CHILL YOUR BODY, NOT YOUR SASS

DITCH THE HEAT, KEEP THE FLAVOR – RECIPES THAT GET YOU GLOWIN' (NOT OVERHEATIN')

DELPHINE O. LIPPS

© 2025 by Delphine Lipps

All rights reserved. No part of this publication may be reproduced, distributed, or transmitted in any form or by any means, including photocopying, recording, or other electronic or mechanical methods, without the prior written permission of the publisher, except in the case of brief quotations embodied in critical reviews and certain other noncommercial uses permitted by copyright law.

Contents

Preface...6

THE SCIENCE OF INFLAMMATION 7

THE MODERN INFLAMMATORY STORM 13

NUTRIGENOMICS OF INFLAMMATION 24

METABOLIC FLEXIBILITY AND INFLAMMATORY ADAPTATION 35

YOUR GUT'S SECRET CONTROL CENTER 48

CORE PRINCIPLES OF ANTI-INFLAMMATORY EATING 58

STRESS MANAGEMENT AND INFLAMMATION 69

ENVIRONMENTAL DETOXIFICATION 81

Breakfast Recipes 93

Lunch and Dinner Options 109

Snacks and Treats 124

Soups and Stews 135

Low FODMAP Options 146

Beverages and Liquid Diet Options 157

30 Days Meal Plan 166

Recipe Index 172

Preface

If you're reading this, chances are you're tired of feeling tired. You've likely been told your blood work is "normal" while you struggle with symptoms that make each day feel like an uphill battle. You're not alone, and more importantly, you're not imagining it.

We are living through the largest health crisis in human history—one that hides in plain sight. While we've conquered many infectious diseases and extended human lifespan, we've simultaneously created an epidemic of chronic inflammatory conditions that didn't exist in our ancestors.

Consider these sobering statistics:

- The Numbers Tell the Story:
- 6 in 10 American adults have at least one chronic disease driven by inflammation
- 133 million Americans—nearly half the population—live with conditions like diabetes, heart disease, arthritis, and autoimmune disorders
- Healthcare spending on chronic inflammatory diseases exceeds $3.8 trillion annually
- The average American takes 4 prescription medications daily, many to manage inflammatory conditions
- Autoimmune diseases alone affect 50 million Americans—more than cancer and heart disease combined

- The Modern Paradox:
- We have access to more medical technology than ever, yet chronic disease rates continue climbing
- We spend more on healthcare per capita than any other nation, yet rank 46th in life expectancy
- Depression and anxiety rates have tripled in the past decade, largely due to inflammatory brain changes
- 1 in 3 children now develops allergies or asthma—conditions virtually unknown 100 years ago

What Changed?

The answer lies in a fundamental mismatch between our ancient biology and our modern environment. In just 150 years—a blink of an eye in evolutionary terms—we've radically transformed how we eat, move, sleep, work, and live. Our immune systems, designed to protect us from acute threats, now face chronic challenges they were never meant to handle.

- The Perfect Storm:
- We consume 152 pounds of sugar per person annually (compared to 4 pounds in 1700)
- 73% of the food supply is ultra-processed, containing ingredients our bodies don't recognize
- The average person encounters over 700 different chemicals daily
- We sit for 9+ hours daily, moving less than our ancestors did in a single morning
- Sleep deprivation affects 70% of adults regularly
- Stress has become so common we consider it normal

The result? Our protective inflammatory system—designed to save us—has become our greatest health threat.

The Research Revolution

Over the past two decades, groundbreaking research has revealed that chronic inflammation is the common thread connecting most modern diseases. Scientists now understand that conditions as diverse as heart disease, diabetes, Alzheimer's, depression, arthritis, and even cancer share this fundamental inflammatory root.

This discovery changes everything. Instead of treating each condition separately, we can address the underlying inflammatory patterns that drive multiple health problems simultaneously.

- The Evidence is Overwhelming:
- Harvard's landmark studies following over 200,000 people for 30+ years show that anti-inflammatory diets reduce disease risk by 20-40%

- The PREDIMED study demonstrated that Mediterranean-style eating prevents heart attacks and strokes better than low-fat diets
- Research from leading institutions confirms that lifestyle interventions can reverse inflammatory biomarkers within days to weeks
- Studies show that simple dietary changes can be as effective as medications for many inflammatory conditions

Why I Wrote This Book

As a food researcher who has spent over two decades studying the intersection of nutrition and inflammation, I've witnessed both the devastating impact of our modern inflammatory crisis and the remarkable healing capacity of the human body when given the right support.

I've watched people transform their lives—not through complex medical interventions or expensive treatments, but through understanding and working with their body's natural healing systems. I've seen chronic pain disappear, energy levels soar, brain fog lift, and "incurable" conditions improve dramatically when people learn to reduce their inflammatory burden.

But here's what frustrates me: this information remains scattered across thousands of research papers, hidden behind medical jargon, and often contradicted by well-meaning but outdated dietary advice. Meanwhile, millions of people suffer needlessly from conditions that could be prevented or significantly improved through anti-inflammatory living.

What Makes This Book Different

This isn't another diet book promising quick fixes. It's a comprehensive guide based on the latest science, translated into practical strategies you can implement immediately. You'll discover:

- Evidence-Based Solutions: Every recommendation is backed by peer-reviewed research, not food fads or marketing claims.
- Personalized Approaches: Because one size doesn't fit all, you'll learn to tailor anti-inflammatory strategies to your unique biology, preferences, and circumstances.
- Immediate Action Steps: Each chapter includes practical tools you can use right away, so you don't have to wait until you finish reading to start feeling better.
- Whole-Life Integration: True healing goes beyond food. You'll learn how stress, sleep, movement, and environment all contribute to inflammatory health.
- Real-World Application: This book is written for busy, real people dealing with real challenges—not for those with unlimited time and resources.

A Personal Note

If you're skeptical, I understand. You may have tried other approaches that didn't work. You may feel overwhelmed by conflicting health information. You may wonder if real change is possible for you.

I want you to know that your body is not broken. Your symptoms are not character flaws or signs of weakness. They're your body's way of communicating that it needs support. When you learn to listen to these signals and respond appropriately, healing happens naturally.

The strategies in this book have been tested not just in research laboratories, but in real kitchens, by real people, living real lives. They work because they're based on supporting your body's existing wisdom rather than fighting against it.

Your journey to vibrant health doesn't require perfection—it requires knowledge, intention, and consistent small actions. You already have everything you need to begin. This book will show you how.

PART I

UNDERSTANDING INFLAMMATION

Chapter 1

The Science of Inflammation

> Inflammation is not your enemy—it's your body's way of protecting you. But like a smoke alarm that won't stop beeping, sometimes this protective system gets stuck in the 'on' position.

Imagine your body as a well-organized city with its own emergency response system. When danger strikes—whether it's a cut on your finger, a virus trying to invade, or harmful bacteria attempting to set up camp—your body's "fire department" springs into action. This emergency response is called inflammation, and it's one of the most important protective mechanisms you have.

But here's where things get interesting: this same system that's designed to heal and protect you can sometimes become your biggest health challenge. Let me explain how this works and why understanding it could be the key to transforming your health.

Acute Inflammation: Your Body's Superhero Response

Think of acute inflammation as your body's superhero team rushing to save the day. When you cut your finger, twist your ankle, or catch a cold, this is exactly what you want to happen:

*The Scene: You accidentally cut your finger while chopping vegetables.

*What Happens Next: Within seconds, your body launches a coordinated rescue mission:
- Blood vessels widen to rush more immune cells to the injury site
- The area becomes red and warm (that's increased blood flow bringing help)
- Swelling occurs (your body's way of diluting toxins and bringing more resources)
- Pain signals fire (nature's way of making you protect the injured area)
- Healing cells arrive and begin repair work

This entire process usually lasts hours to days, and then—here's the key—it turns off. The swelling goes down, the redness fades, and your finger heals. Mission accomplished. This is inflammation working perfectly.

Chronic Inflammation: When the Fire Alarm Won't Stop

Now imagine your smoke alarm started beeping at 2 AM, but instead of a real fire, it was just triggered by steam from your shower. You'd want to turn it off, right? But what if it kept beeping... for months... or years?

This is chronic inflammation. Your body's emergency response system gets triggered by things like:
- Processed foods that your body sees as "foreign invaders"
- Chronic stress that never lets your system calm down
- Environmental toxins that constantly irritate your cells
- Poor sleep that prevents your body from completing its natural healing cycles

- Lack of movement that allows inflammatory chemicals to build up

Unlike acute inflammation that comes and goes, chronic inflammation is like having a low-grade fever that never breaks. It's subtle, often silent, but it's constantly wearing down your body's systems.

Here's what makes chronic inflammation so dangerous: It doesn't just affect one area—it travels throughout your entire body via your bloodstream, affecting organs and systems that seemed completely unrelated to the original problem.

THE INFLAMMATORY CASCADE: YOUR BODY'S CHEMICAL CONVERSATION

I know "biochemical pathways" sounds intimidating, but think of it as your body's internal communication system—like a group chat where your cells are constantly sending messages to each other.

The Message System That Runs Your Body

When your body detects a threat, it starts what scientists call the "inflammatory cascade." Imagine it like this:

- ❖ Step 1: The Alert: Your cells act like neighborhood watchdogs. When they spot trouble (damaged tissue, harmful bacteria, or irritating chemicals), they immediately send out an alarm signal.

- ❖ Step 2: The Messengers: These alarm signals are carried by special chemical messengers with complex names, but you can think of them as your body's internal postal service:

  - Cytokines: Think of these as urgent text messages between your cells. Some say "Send help immediately!" while others later say "All clear, stand down."
  - Prostaglandins: These are like volume controls for your inflammatory response. Some turn up the heat (causing pain and swelling), while others turn it down (promoting healing and resolution).
  - Histamines: You might know these from allergy medications. They're like the emergency broadcast system, quickly spreading the alert throughout your body.

- ❖ Step 3: The Response Team: Once the messages are sent, your body's response team kicks into gear:
  - White blood cells rush to the scene like paramedics
  - Blood vessels change their behavior to help or hinder different substances
  - Specialized cleanup crews arrive to remove damaged tissue and debris
  - Repair workers start rebuilding and healing

When the Conversation Goes Wrong

In chronic inflammation, it's like your body's group chat gets stuck in an endless loop of emergency messages. The "all clear" signal never comes, so the conversation keeps escalating. This constant chatter of inflammatory messages affects every system in your body.

THE HIDDEN TRIGGERS: HOW MODERN LIFE HIJACKS YOUR IMMUNE SYSTEM

Your inflammatory system evolved over millions of years to handle specific threats: injuries, infections, and toxic plants. But in the last 100 years, we've introduced challenges your body has never seen before.

The Modern Inflammatory Storm

- Processed Foods: Your immune system doesn't recognize many chemicals in processed foods. When you eat something with 20 ingredients you can't pronounce, your body treats it like a foreign invader and mounts an inflammatory response.

*Real Example: Jeanette, a busy mom, ate fast food for lunch daily. She couldn't understand why she always felt tired and achy in the afternoons. When she switched to homemade meals for just two weeks, her energy levels soared and her joint pain disappeared.

- Chronic Stress: Your ancestors faced acute stress (like running from a lion) followed by long periods of calm. Modern stress is different—it's constant, low-level, and never-ending. Your body stays in fight-or-flight mode, continuously pumping out stress hormones that fuel inflammation.

- Sleep Disruption: Think of sleep as your body's nightly maintenance shift. During quality sleep, your body produces powerful anti-inflammatory compounds and clears out inflammatory waste products. Poor sleep is like skipping this crucial cleanup time.

- Sedentary Lifestyle: Movement acts like a natural anti-inflammatory medicine. When you sit for hours, inflammatory chemicals build up in your system like stagnant water. Regular movement keeps these chemicals flowing and helps your body process them efficiently.

- Environmental Toxins: From air pollution to household chemicals, your body is constantly exposed to substances that trigger inflammatory responses. While you can't avoid everything, awareness helps you make better choices.

HOW INFLAMMATION SHOWS UP IN DAILY LIFE

Let me share some real examples of how chronic inflammation affects people just like you:

Case Study 1: The Executive's Wake-Up Call

Meet David, 45, Marketing Executive

David thought his daily headaches, afternoon energy crashes, and weekend joint pain were just part of getting older. His doctor said his blood work was "normal," but David felt anything but normal.

- ❖ The Hidden Inflammation: David's routine included:
  - Skipping breakfast, then drinking 4 cups of coffee
  - Fast food lunches eaten at his desk
  - High-stress meetings with no breaks
  - Staying up late answering emails
  - Weekend "recovery" sessions with alcohol and takeout

*The Turning Point: When David started tracking his symptoms alongside his food and stress levels, he noticed clear patterns. His worst days always followed his highest-stress, poorest-eating days.

- ❖ The Transformation: Within 30 days of following an anti-inflammatory approach:
  - Headaches reduced from daily to occasional
  - Energy levels stabilized throughout the day
  - Joint pain disappeared completely
  - Sleep quality improved dramatically
  - Work performance actually increased despite spending less time at his desk

Case Study 2: The Mother's Discovery

Meet Lisa, 38, Stay-at-Home Mom

Lisa struggled with what she called "mystery symptoms"—fatigue, mood swings, digestive issues, and frequent colds. Multiple doctors couldn't find anything wrong, leaving her feeling frustrated and dismissed.

❖ The Hidden Inflammation: Lisa's challenges included:
- Emotional eating when stressed with kids
- Relying on processed snacks for quick energy
- Interrupted sleep from night wakings
- Constant low-level stress from managing household chaos
- Putting everyone else's needs before her own

*The Realization: Lisa discovered that her symptoms weren't separate problems—they were all connected through chronic inflammation. Her body was constantly in emergency mode, never getting a chance to rest and repair.

❖ The Healing: By addressing inflammation through:
- Simple, whole-food meals (not perfect, just better)
- 10-minute daily walks outside
- A consistent bedtime routine
- Stress-reduction techniques she could do with kids around

Lisa's energy returned, her mood stabilized, and she stopped getting sick every month. Most importantly, she felt like herself again.

Case Study 3: The Athlete's Plateau

Meet Marcus, 28, Weekend Warrior

Marcus exercised regularly and ate what he thought was a healthy diet, but he couldn't shake nagging injuries, slow recovery times, and performance plateaus.

❖ The Hidden Inflammation: Despite his active lifestyle, Marcus had:
- A diet high in inflammatory foods (sports drinks, protein bars, processed "health" foods)
- Inadequate recovery time between workouts
- Chronic stress from work that prevented proper healing
- Poor sleep quality despite feeling tired

❖ The Breakthrough: When Marcus shifted focus from just exercise to overall anti-inflammatory living:
- His chronic shoulder pain resolved
- Recovery time between workouts shortened dramatically
- Performance improvements resumed
- Sleep quality improved, leading to better training sessions

The Inflammation-Disease Connection: Why This Matters for Your Future

Chronic inflammation isn't just about feeling tired or achy today—it's about your long-term health. Research shows that chronic inflammation is involved in nearly every major disease:

- Heart Disease: Inflammation damages blood vessel walls, leading to plaque buildup and heart attacks.
- Diabetes: Inflammatory chemicals interfere with insulin function, making blood sugar control difficult.
- Cancer: Chronic inflammation creates an environment where cancer cells can grow and spread more easily.
- Alzheimer's Disease: Brain inflammation contributes to the death of brain cells and memory loss.
- Arthritis: Inflammatory chemicals attack joint tissue, causing pain and deterioration.
- Depression: Inflammatory signals directly affect brain chemistry and mood regulation.

But here's the hopeful truth: because these diseases share the common thread of chronic inflammation, addressing inflammation can help prevent or improve multiple health conditions simultaneously.

Your Inflammation Reality Check

Take a moment to honestly assess your current inflammatory load. Do any of these sound familiar?

❖ Daily Symptoms Checklist:
- Fatigue that doesn't improve with rest
- Frequent headaches or brain fog
- Digestive issues (bloating, gas, irregular bowel movements)
- Mood swings or irritability
- Frequent colds or infections
- Aches and pains with no clear cause
- Difficulty losing weight despite efforts
- Poor sleep quality
- Slow healing from minor injuries
- Skin problems (acne, eczema, rashes)

If you checked several items, you're likely dealing with chronic inflammation. But don't worry—recognizing this is the first step toward healing.

The Path Forward: Your Body's Incredible Healing Capacity

Here's the most important thing I want you to understand: your body wants to heal. Given the right conditions, your inflammatory system can return to its natural, balanced state remarkably quickly.

I've seen people experience significant improvements in:
- 3-7 days: Better energy and mood
- 1-2 weeks: Improved digestion and sleep
- 3-4 weeks: Reduced pain and clearer thinking
- 2-3 months: Significant changes in lab markers and chronic symptoms

Your body isn't broken—it's just responding to the environment you've created for it. Change the environment, and you change the response.

What You Can Start Today

While we'll dive deep into specific strategies in later chapters, here are three simple steps you can take right now:

1. Add Color to Your Next Meal: Include one colorful vegetable or fruit you don't normally eat. The natural compounds that create these colors are powerful anti-inflammatory agents.

2. Take Three Deep Breaths: When you feel stressed, take three slow, deep breaths. This simple act switches your nervous system from inflammatory stress mode to healing rest mode.

3. Move for Two Minutes: Stand up, stretch, or take a short walk. Movement helps flush inflammatory chemicals from your system and promotes healing circulation.

These might seem too simple to matter, but remember—chronic inflammation develops from small, repeated exposures to inflammatory triggers. Healing happens the same way: small, repeated actions that support your body's natural anti-inflammatory processes.

The body benefits from movement, and the mind benefits from stillness. But both benefit most from understanding.

Chapter 1 Key Takeaways

❖ What You Learned:
- Inflammation is your body's protective response that can become problematic when it doesn't turn off
- Chronic inflammation affects every system in your body through chemical messengers
- Modern lifestyle factors constantly trigger your inflammatory system
- Your gut and brain communicate directly through inflammatory pathways
- Most chronic diseases share chronic inflammation as a common factor

❖ What You Can Do Right Now:
- Start noticing patterns between your symptoms and lifestyle factors
- Add one colorful, whole food to your next meal
- Practice three deep breaths when stressed
- Take movement breaks every hour
- Begin viewing symptoms as your body's way of communicating its needs

Chapter 2

The Modern Inflammatory Storm

Your body is designed to thrive, but it's operating in an environment it was never designed for. Understanding this mismatch is the first step to reclaiming your health.

Imagine if you took a person from 1900 and transported them to today. They'd be amazed by our technology, medical advances, and convenience. But their body would be overwhelmed by something they couldn't see: the constant inflammatory assault of modern living.

Here's the startling truth: in just over 100 years, we've fundamentally changed almost everything about how humans live, while our biology has remained essentially the same. Your body is still operating with the same inflammatory system your great-great-grandmother had, but it's now trying to cope with challenges that didn't exist even 50 years ago.

This chapter will help you understand why you might be struggling with symptoms that seem to come out of nowhere, why "eating healthy" according to conventional wisdom might not be working for you, and most importantly, how to navigate this modern world in a way that supports rather than sabotages your body's natural healing abilities.

THE INVISIBLE ENEMY: ENVIRONMENTAL TOXINS AND YOUR INFLAMMATORY BURDEN

Every single day, your body encounters thousands of chemicals that didn't exist when your immune system was developing. Think of your liver and immune system as an overwhelmed security team at a concert venue—they're working overtime to screen out potential threats, but the crowd keeps getting bigger and more complex.

- ❖ The Numbers Are Staggering:
- The average person is exposed to over 700 different chemicals daily
- Your blood contains traces of at least 200 industrial chemicals
- Many of these chemicals are stored in your fat tissue for years or decades
- Your body treats many of these foreign substances as invaders, triggering inflammatory responses

Where These Hidden Triggers Hide

- ❖ In Your Home:

Nina's Story: Nina couldn't figure out why she woke up every morning with a stuffy nose and headache. She ate well, exercised, and got enough sleep. The culprit? The "fresh linen" air fresheners plugged into every room and the fabric softener she'd been using for years. Within a week of removing these, her morning symptoms disappeared.

- ❖ Common household inflammatory triggers include:

- Air fresheners and scented candles (synthetic fragrances)
- Cleaning products with harsh chemicals
- Non-stick cookware releasing toxic compounds when heated
- Carpets and furniture treated with flame retardants
- Personal care products with endocrine-disrupting chemicals

❖ In Your Water:

Your tap water might look clean, but it often contains:
- Chlorine and chloramine (added for disinfection but inflammatory to your gut)
- Heavy metals like lead and mercury
- Pharmaceutical residues from medications
- Industrial chemicals and pesticide runoff

Simple Fix: Installing a quality water filter was one of the best investments Maria ever made. Not only did her digestive issues improve, but her skin cleared up and her energy increased. "I didn't realize how much inflammation was coming from something as basic as my drinking water," she said.

❖ In Your Food (Beyond the Obvious):

Even foods labeled as "natural" can carry inflammatory burdens:
- Pesticide residues on fruits and vegetables
- Antibiotics and hormones in conventionally raised meat
- Heavy metals in certain fish
- Mold toxins in coffee, nuts, and grains
- Plastic packaging chemicals that leach into food

Your Body's Overwhelmed Detox System

Think of your liver as your body's main water treatment plant. When it's working properly, it can handle a reasonable amount of toxins. But when it's overwhelmed—like a treatment plant during a flood—toxins back up into your system, triggering widespread inflammation.

❖ Signs Your Detox System Is Overwhelmed:
- Fatigue that doesn't improve with rest
- Skin problems (acne, rashes, eczema)
- Chemical sensitivities that seem to get worse over time
- Brain fog and difficulty concentrating
- Digestive issues and bloating
- Frequent headaches
- Difficulty losing weight despite healthy eating and exercise

The Good News: Your body has an incredible capacity to heal and detoxify when given the right support. Small changes in reducing your toxic load can yield big improvements in how you feel.

THE PROCESSED FOOD TRAP: HOW THE FOOD INDUSTRY CREATES INFLAMMATORY CHAOS

We're living through the largest uncontrolled experiment in human history. In just 70 years, we've gone from eating foods our bodies recognize to consuming products our immune systems treat as foreign invaders.

❖ The Transformation Timeline:
- 1950s: Most food was whole, local, and seasonal
- 1960s-70s: Processed convenience foods became mainstream

- 1980s-90s: Low-fat, high-sugar processed foods dominated
- 2000s-2010s: Ultra-processed foods became 60% of the American diet
- Today: The average grocery store contains over 40,000 products, most containing inflammatory ingredients

The Inflammatory Ingredient Hall of Shame

- ❖ High-Fructose Corn Syrup (HFCS): Your liver processes HFCS differently than natural sugars, creating inflammatory byproducts and contributing to fatty liver disease. It's hidden in:
- Soft drinks and fruit juices
- Bread and crackers
- Salad dressings and condiments
- Yogurt and "healthy" snacks

Real Example: When Tom eliminated HFCS from his diet, his afternoon energy crashes disappeared, and he lost 15 pounds without changing anything else. "I had no idea how much this one ingredient was affecting me," he said.

- ❖ Trans Fats and Damaged Oils: These aren't just unhealthy—they're actively inflammatory. They're found in:
- Fried foods from restaurants
- Packaged baked goods
- Margarine and vegetable shortening
- Many processed snacks

- ❖ Artificial Additives: Your immune system doesn't recognize these synthetic chemicals:
- Artificial colors (linked to hyperactivity and inflammation)
- Preservatives like BHT and BHA
- Flavor enhancers like MSG
- Artificial sweeteners that disrupt gut bacteria

Refined Sugars: Sugar doesn't just cause blood sugar spikes—it directly triggers inflammatory pathways. The average American consumes 152 pounds of sugar per year, compared to 4 pounds in 1700.

The Marketing Deception

Health Halo Foods: Foods marketed as healthy but loaded with inflammatory ingredients:
- Granola bars with 15+ grams of sugar
- "Whole grain" breads with high-fructose corn syrup
- Flavored yogurts with artificial colors and flavors
- Sports drinks with synthetic dyes and excessive sugar
- "Natural" foods with natural flavors (which can contain hundreds of chemical compounds)

Lisa's Awakening: Lisa thought she was eating healthy by choosing products labeled "organic," "natural," and "whole grain." When she started reading ingredient lists instead of marketing claims, she realized many of her "healthy" choices contained 10-20 ingredients she couldn't pronounce. Switching to truly simple foods transformed her energy levels within days.

The Addiction Factor

Processed foods are literally designed to be addictive. Food scientists create what they call the "bliss point"—the perfect combination of sugar, salt, and fat that triggers pleasure centers in your brain while leaving you wanting more.

This creates a vicious cycle:
1. You eat processed food
2. It triggers inflammation and blood sugar spikes
3. You crash and crave more processed food
4. You eat more, perpetuating the cycle
5. Chronic inflammation develops

Breaking the Cycle: Understanding this isn't about willpower—it's about biology. When you stabilize your blood sugar and reduce inflammatory foods, the cravings naturally diminish.

THE STRESS-SLEEP-INFLAMMATION TRIANGLE

Chronic Stress: Your Body's False Emergency

Your stress response system evolved for acute threats—like escaping from a predator. But modern stress is different: it's chronic, psychological, and never-ending.

- ❖ Modern Stress Triggers:
- Work deadlines and job insecurity
- Financial pressures
- Relationship conflicts
- Social media comparison
- News and information overload
- Traffic and commuting
- Parenting pressures
- Caring for aging parents

- ❖ How Chronic Stress Fuels Inflammation:

When you're stressed, your body releases cortisol and adrenaline. In short bursts, these hormones are helpful. But when they're constantly elevated:
- They suppress your immune system's ability to turn off inflammation
- They increase production of inflammatory chemicals
- They disrupt your gut bacteria balance
- They interfere with sleep and recovery processes
- They promote storage of inflammatory belly fat

David's Reality: David, a project manager, lived in constant low-level panic about deadlines. He'd wake up thinking about work, check emails during meals, and fall asleep scrolling through work messages. His body was stuck in emergency mode 24/7. Within a month of implementing stress-management techniques, his chronic back pain—which doctors couldn't explain—completely disappeared.

Sleep Deprivation: The Inflammation Multiplier

Sleep isn't just rest—it's when your body performs critical anti-inflammatory maintenance. Think of sleep as your body's nightly cleanup crew.

- ❖ What Happens During Quality Sleep:
- Your brain clears out inflammatory waste products
- Your body produces powerful anti-inflammatory compounds
- Your gut bacteria rebalance themselves
- Your stress hormones reset to healthy levels

- Your immune system calibrates itself for the next day

❖ How Poor Sleep Fuels Inflammation:
- Even one night of poor sleep increases inflammatory markers
- Sleep deprivation makes you more sensitive to pain
- Your body produces more stress hormones when sleep-deprived
- Your gut becomes more permeable, allowing inflammatory toxins into your bloodstream
- Your appetite hormones get disrupted, leading to inflammatory food cravings

❖ The Modern Sleep Disruptors:
- Blue light from screens interfering with melatonin production
- Caffeine consumed too late in the day
- Irregular sleep schedules disrupting circadian rhythms
- Bedroom environments that are too warm, bright, or noisy
- Stress and racing thoughts preventing deep sleep
- Alcohol, which fragments sleep despite making you feel drowsy

Maria's Transformation: Maria was caught in a vicious cycle—stress from work caused poor sleep, which made her more stressed and craving inflammatory foods. When she committed to a consistent bedtime routine and removed screens from her bedroom, not only did her sleep improve, but her anxiety decreased and her chronic digestive issues resolved.

The Stress-Sleep-Inflammation Downward Spiral

Here's how these factors feed off each other:
1. Chronic stress disrupts sleep quality
2. Poor sleep increases stress hormones and inflammation
3. Inflammation makes you more sensitive to stress
4. Increased stress sensitivity disrupts sleep further
5. The cycle continues, getting worse over time

Breaking the Cycle: The good news is that improving any one factor helps the others. Better sleep reduces stress sensitivity. Stress management improves sleep quality. Both reduce inflammation.

THE SITTING DISEASE: HOW SEDENTARY LIVING INFLAMES YOUR BODY

Your ancestors moved constantly—hunting, gathering, farming, walking everywhere. Movement wasn't exercise; it was life. Your circulatory, lymphatic, and immune systems all depend on regular movement to function properly.

❖ The Modern Movement Crisis:
- The average office worker sits 10 hours per day
- Many people move less than 30 minutes total per day
- We've replaced physical activity with mental activity
- Even people who exercise regularly may sit for most of their waking hours

How Sitting Fuels Inflammation

- Stagnant Circulation: When you sit for hours, inflammatory chemicals build up in your bloodstream like stagnant water in a pond. Movement acts like a flowing river, keeping these chemicals moving and helping your body process them.

- Muscle Deactivation: Your muscles produce anti-inflammatory compounds when they contract. When you're sedentary, you lose this natural anti-inflammatory medicine.

- Metabolic Disruption: Prolonged sitting disrupts your body's ability to regulate blood sugar and fat metabolism, leading to inflammatory metabolic syndrome.

- Lymphatic Stagnation: Your lymphatic system (your body's waste removal system) doesn't have a pump like your heart. It relies on muscle contractions to move lymph fluid. Without movement, inflammatory waste products accumulate.

Mike's Discovery: Mike worked at a computer for 8-10 hours daily. Despite eating well and exercising 30 minutes in the morning, he struggled with afternoon fatigue, brain fog, and chronic lower back pain. When he started taking 2-minute movement breaks every hour, his symptoms dramatically improved. "I couldn't believe such a simple change made such a big difference," he said.

The Exercise Paradox

Here's something surprising: you can't out-exercise a sedentary lifestyle. Even if you work out intensely for an hour, sitting for the remaining 15 waking hours still promotes inflammation.

The Solution: It's not about perfect workouts—it's about consistent movement throughout the day. Research shows that breaking up sitting time with just 2-3 minutes of light movement every hour is more beneficial than one long workout session.

- ❖ Simple Movement Solutions:
- Stand during phone calls
- Walk while thinking through problems
- Take the stairs instead of elevators
- Park farther away or get off transit one stop early
- Set hourly movement reminders
- Have walking meetings when possible
- Do basic stretches or exercises during TV commercial breaks

THE MICROBIOME DISRUPTION EPIDEMIC

You're not just human—you're a walking ecosystem. Your body contains trillions of bacteria, viruses, and other microorganisms that play crucial roles in your health. These microscopic partners help:
- Digest your food and produce essential nutrients
- Regulate your immune system and inflammation levels
- Protect you from harmful pathogens
- Communicate with your brain and influence your mood
- Control your metabolism and weight

The Great Microbiome Destruction

In just a few generations, we've decimated the microbial diversity that humans carried for millennia:

- ❖ The Main Culprits:
- Antibiotics: While life-saving when needed, they're often overprescribed and kill beneficial bacteria along with harmful ones
- Processed Foods: Feed harmful bacteria while starving beneficial ones

- Chemical Exposure: Pesticides, preservatives, and household chemicals disrupt microbial balance
- Chronic Stress: Stress hormones directly impact gut bacteria composition
- Lack of Fiber: Beneficial bacteria need fiber to survive and thrive
- Over-Sanitization: While hygiene is important, excessive use of antibacterial products reduces microbial diversity

When Your Microbiome Goes Wrong

❖ Dysbiosis (microbial imbalance) creates a cascade of inflammatory problems:
- Increased intestinal permeability ("leaky gut")
- Systemic inflammation as bacterial toxins enter your bloodstream
- Impaired immune function and increased infections
- Mood disorders as gut bacteria influence brain chemistry
- Digestive issues and food sensitivities
- Difficulty maintaining healthy weight
- Increased risk of autoimmune conditions

Jennifer's Journey: Jennifer had taken multiple rounds of antibiotics for recurring infections. Afterward, she developed severe digestive issues, frequent colds, anxiety, and brain fog. When she focused on rebuilding her microbiome through fermented foods and prebiotic fiber, her symptoms gradually resolved. "I didn't realize how connected my gut health was to everything else," she reflected.

The Microbiome-Inflammation Connection

Your gut bacteria are like internal peacekeepers. Beneficial bacteria:
- Produce anti-inflammatory compounds
- Train your immune system to respond appropriately
- Maintain the gut barrier to prevent inflammatory toxins from entering your bloodstream
- Compete with harmful bacteria for space and resources

When harmful bacteria dominate:
- They produce inflammatory toxins
- They damage your gut lining
- They trigger inappropriate immune responses
- They create cravings for foods that feed them (usually sugar and processed foods)

SOCIAL DETERMINANTS: THE HIDDEN HEALTH INEQUALITY

While personal choices matter enormously, it's important to recognize that not everyone has equal access to anti-inflammatory living. Your zip code can be more predictive of your health than your genetic code.

❖ Environmental Justice Issues:
- Low-income neighborhoods often have higher pollution levels
- Food deserts make fresh, whole foods difficult to access
- Unsafe neighborhoods limit opportunities for outdoor exercise
- Work schedules may not allow time for meal preparation
- Chronic financial stress creates persistent inflammatory responses

❖ The Inequality-Inflammation Connection:
- Chronic stress from financial insecurity elevates cortisol levels
- Poor air quality in certain areas increases respiratory inflammation
- Limited access to healthcare means inflammatory conditions go untreated

- Social isolation and discrimination create chronic stress responses
- Shift work disrupts circadian rhythms and sleep quality

Building Community Solutions

❖ What You Can Do:
- Support local farmers markets and community gardens
- Advocate for cleaner air and water in your community
- Share knowledge and resources with neighbors
- Create walking groups or community exercise programs
- Support policies that improve environmental health for everyone

Community Success Story: In Oakland, California, a group of residents noticed high rates of asthma and diabetes in their neighborhood. They organized to create community gardens, walking groups, and healthy cooking classes. Over five years, they documented significant improvements in community health markers and stronger social connections.

THE COMPOUND EFFECT: WHEN EVERYTHING ADDS UP

Why Small Exposures Matter

You might think, "A little artificial color won't hurt me" or "One missed night of sleep isn't a big deal." And you'd be right—if these were isolated incidents. But the reality is that modern life creates a compound inflammatory burden.

The Inflammatory Load Equation: Daily toxin exposure + processed food consumption + chronic stress + poor sleep + sedentary lifestyle + disrupted microbiome + social stressors = Chronic inflammatory overload

It's not any one factor that's the problem—it's the cumulative effect of all these factors operating simultaneously.

The Tipping Point: Your body can often handle some inflammatory stress. But there's a tipping point where your anti-inflammatory systems become overwhelmed. That's when symptoms appear, seemingly out of nowhere.

Rachel's Realization: Rachel couldn't understand why she suddenly developed joint pain, fatigue, and digestive issues at age 35. "I've always been healthy," she said. When we mapped out her lifestyle changes over the previous two years—new stressful job, irregular sleep from night shifts, more takeout food, less time for exercise, plus moving to a more polluted area—the compound effect became clear. Addressing these factors systematically restored her health.

The Positive Compound Effect

Here's the hopeful flip side: just as negative factors compound to create inflammation, positive factors compound to create healing. Small, consistent improvements in multiple areas can yield dramatic results.

The Healing Equation: Reduced toxic load + anti-inflammatory foods + stress management + quality sleep + regular movement + healthy microbiome + social support = Exponential healing

Your Personal Inflammatory Storm Assessment

Take a moment to honestly evaluate your current inflammatory load. Rate each area from 1-5 (1 = very low inflammatory burden, 5 = very high inflammatory burden):

- ❖ Environmental Toxins (___/5):
- Use of conventional cleaning and personal care products
- Air quality in your home and work environment
- Water quality and filtration
- Exposure to chemicals and pollution

- ❖ Food Quality (___/5):
- Frequency of processed food consumption
- Amount of sugar and refined foods in your diet
- Exposure to pesticides and food additives
- Reliance on packaged vs. fresh foods

- ❖ Stress Level (___/5):
- Chronic work or life stress
- Lack of stress management techniques
- Feeling overwhelmed or anxious regularly
- Poor work-life balance

- ❖ Sleep Quality (___/5):
- Irregular sleep schedule
- Poor sleep environment
- Difficulty falling or staying asleep
- Feeling unrefreshed despite adequate sleep time

- ❖ Movement Patterns (___/5):
- Hours spent sitting daily
- Lack of regular physical activity
- Sedentary work environment
- Limited recreational movement

- ❖ Microbiome Health (___/5):
- Recent antibiotic use
- Low fiber intake
- Frequent digestive issues
- Limited fermented food consumption

- ❖ Social Factors (___/5):
- Financial or housing stress
- Limited social support
- Exposure to discrimination or trauma
- Unsafe or unhealthy living environment

Total Score: ___/35

- ❖ Interpreting Your Score:
- 7-14: Low inflammatory burden—focus on maintenance and prevention
- 15-21: Moderate inflammatory burden—targeted improvements will yield significant benefits
- 22-28: High inflammatory burden—systematic changes across multiple areas recommended
- 29-35: Very high inflammatory burden—consider working with healthcare practitioners while implementing changes

What you need is awareness, intention, and consistent small actions that support your body's natural healing processes.

Where to Start

Based on working with thousands of people, here are the most impactful changes to prioritize:

1. Sleep Quality: This affects everything else. Poor sleep makes every other inflammatory factor worse.

2. Food Quality: Focus on whole foods over processed ones. This single change addresses multiple inflammatory pathways.

3. Movement: Regular, gentle movement throughout the day beats sporadic intense exercise.

4. Stress Management: Find techniques that work for your lifestyle and practice them consistently.

5. Environmental Cleanup: Start with simple swaps in products you use daily.

Your Anti-Inflammatory Mindset Shift

Instead of thinking about what you need to eliminate, think about what you can add:
- Add more colorful vegetables instead of just removing processed foods
- Add movement breaks instead of just sitting less
- Add stress-relief activities instead of just avoiding stress
- Add beneficial bacteria instead of just killing harmful ones

This positive approach makes change feel empowering rather than restrictive.

Hope in the Storm

Yes, we're living in challenging times for human health. But we're also living in times of incredible knowledge and opportunity. You have access to information and choices that previous generations never had.

Every day, you make dozens of choices that either contribute to inflammation or support healing. Now that you understand the landscape, you can make these choices consciously and strategically.

Remember: your body wants to heal. Your immune system wants to function properly. Your energy wants to be stable. Your mood wants to be balanced. When you remove the barriers and provide the right support, healing happens naturally.

You can't control every aspect of the modern world, but you can control how you respond to it. That response makes all the difference.

Chapter 2 Key Takeaways

❖ What You Learned:
- Modern life creates an unprecedented inflammatory burden through multiple pathways

- Environmental toxins, processed foods, chronic stress, poor sleep, sedentary lifestyle, and microbiome disruption all compound to create inflammation
- Social and environmental factors beyond individual control also impact inflammatory health
- The compound effect works both ways—negative factors multiply problems, but positive factors multiply healing

❖ What You Can Do Right Now:
- Assess your personal inflammatory load using the chapter assessment
- Choose one area from your highest-scoring categories to focus on first
- Make one simple swap today (e.g., replace one processed food with a whole food, take movement breaks, or switch to a natural cleaning product)
- Start paying attention to how different factors in your environment affect how you feel

Chapter 3

Nutrigenomics of Inflammation

Your genes are not your destiny—they're your starting point. Understanding how your unique genetic makeup responds to different foods and lifestyle factors is like having a personalized roadmap to optimal health.

Have you ever wondered why your friend can eat pizza and feel fine while it leaves you bloated and tired for days? Or why certain "superfoods" that work miracles for others seem to do nothing for you? The answer lies in your unique genetic code—your personal instruction manual for how your body processes food, handles stress, and manages inflammation.

We're living in an exciting time where cutting-edge genetic science is finally becoming accessible and practical for everyday people like you. This isn't science fiction—it's science fact that you can use starting today to optimize your health in ways that were impossible just a decade ago.

In this chapter, you'll discover how your genes influence your inflammatory responses and, more importantly, how you can work with your genetic blueprint rather than against it. Think of this as upgrading from a one-size-fits-all approach to having a custom-tailored health plan designed specifically for your unique biology.

UNDERSTANDING YOUR GENETIC INFLUENCE ON INFLAMMATION

Genes vs. Genetic Expression: Why You Have More Control Than You Think

First, let's clear up a common misconception. Many people think having certain genes means they're doomed to develop certain health problems. This simply isn't true. Your genes are like light switches—they can be turned on or off by your environment, lifestyle, and food choices.

Here's how it actually works:

- Your Genes: These are like the hardware in your computer—they don't change throughout your life. You inherited them from your parents, and they contain the instructions for making proteins that control various functions in your body.

- Gene Expression: This is like the software running on your computer—it can be updated, modified, and optimized. Gene expression determines whether certain genes are "turned on" (active) or "turned off" (inactive).

- Environmental Triggers: These are like the user inputs that determine which programs run. Your food choices, stress levels, sleep patterns, exercise habits, and even your thoughts can influence which genes get expressed.

Shirley's Story: Shirley discovered she had genetic variants associated with higher inflammation risk. Instead of feeling defeated, she used this information to make targeted dietary changes. Within six months, her inflammatory markers dropped to optimal levels, and she felt better than she had in years. "Knowing my genetic tendencies helped me work with my body instead of against it," she said.

The Inflammation-Gene Connection

Certain genetic variants can influence:
- How efficiently you process different types of fats
- Your body's ability to produce and use antioxidants
- How well you metabolize certain nutrients
- Your sensitivity to inflammatory foods
- Your response to stress and recovery from exercise
- How effectively you detoxify harmful compounds

The key insight: These genetic variants aren't flaws—they're variations that may have provided advantages in different environments. Understanding your variants helps you create the optimal environment for your unique biology.

POE4: THE ALZHEIMER'S GENE THAT'S ACTUALLY ABOUT MUCH MORE

The APOE gene provides instructions for making a protein that helps transport cholesterol and other fats in your bloodstream. There are three main variants: APOE2, APOE3, and APOE4. You inherit one copy from each parent, creating different combinations.

APOE4: The Misunderstood Variant

About 25% of people carry at least one copy of APOE4. While this variant is associated with higher Alzheimer's risk, it's important to understand that:
- Having APOE4 doesn't mean you'll develop Alzheimer's
- Many people with APOE4 never develop cognitive issues
- APOE4 may have provided survival advantages in certain environments
- Understanding your APOE status allows for targeted prevention strategies

Why APOE4 Carriers Need Different Inflammatory Strategies

❖ The APOE4 Difference:
APOE4 carriers tend to:
- Have higher baseline inflammation levels
- Be more sensitive to saturated fats and dietary cholesterol
- Need more aggressive antioxidant support
- Benefit from specific timing of meals and exercise
- Require particular attention to sleep quality and stress management

APOE4-Specific Anti-Inflammatory Protocol

Dietary Strategies for APOE4 Carriers:

❖ Emphasize These Foods:
- Fatty Fish: Wild-caught salmon, sardines, mackerel, and anchovies provide DHA, which is particularly important for APOE4 carriers' brain health

- Colorful Berries: Blueberries, blackberries, and strawberries contain anthocyanins that cross the blood-brain barrier
- Leafy Greens: Spinach, kale, and arugula provide folate and nitrates that support cognitive function
- Nuts and Seeds: Especially walnuts, which provide alpha-linolenic acid (ALA)
- Extra Virgin Olive Oil: Rich in oleocanthal, a natural anti-inflammatory compound
- Turmeric with Black Pepper: The curcumin-piperine combination is particularly beneficial for APOE4 carriers

❖ Foods to Limit or Avoid:
- Saturated Fats from Animal Sources: APOE4 carriers are more sensitive to saturated fat's inflammatory effects
- Processed Meats: Higher inflammatory burden and potential cognitive risks
- Refined Sugars: APOE4 carriers may be more susceptible to glucose-induced inflammation
- Trans Fats: Particularly harmful for brain health in APOE4 carriers
- Excessive Alcohol: APOE4 carriers metabolize alcohol differently and may face higher risks

❖ Meal Timing Strategies:
- Intermittent Fasting: 12-16 hour fasting windows may be particularly beneficial for APOE4 carriers
- Earlier Dinner: Eating dinner at least 3 hours before bed supports better sleep and recovery
- Consistent Meal Timing: Regular eating patterns support circadian rhythm health

Michael's Experience: Michael, an APOE4 carrier, struggled with brain fog and afternoon energy crashes. When he shifted to a lower saturated fat, higher omega-3 diet with intermittent fasting, his cognitive clarity improved dramatically. "I finally feel sharp again," he reported after three months on his personalized protocol.

Lifestyle Modifications for APOE4 Carriers

❖ Exercise Priorities:
- Aerobic Exercise: Particularly important for APOE4 carriers to promote brain-derived neurotrophic factor (BDNF)
- Strength Training: Helps maintain muscle mass and supports healthy aging
- Balance and Coordination: Activities like yoga or tai chi support neuroplasticity

❖ Sleep Optimization:
- APOE4 carriers may need more sleep (8-9 hours) for optimal brain detoxification
- Consistent sleep schedules are crucial for circadian rhythm health
- Sleep position (side sleeping) may help with brain waste clearance

❖ Stress Management:
- Chronic stress may be particularly harmful for APOE4 carriers
- Meditation and mindfulness practices are especially beneficial
- Social connections and community support are crucial for cognitive health

MTHFR: THE METHYLATION MASTER SWITCH

MTHFR stands for methylenetetrahydrofolate reductase—a crucial enzyme that helps your body process folate (vitamin B9) and support methylation. Methylation is like your body's molecular maintenance crew, involved in:
- DNA repair and gene expression
- Neurotransmitter production
- Detoxification processes
- Inflammatory response regulation
- Energy production

Common MTHFR Variants and Their Impact

- ❖ The Two Main Variants:
- C677T: Found in about 40% of people, reduces MTHFR enzyme function by 30-70%
- A1298C: Found in about 30% of people, also reduces enzyme function

You can have zero, one, or two copies of each variant, and the combination affects how well your methylation system works.

Signs Your Methylation System Needs Support

- ❖ Common Symptoms of Poor Methylation:
- Chronic fatigue that doesn't improve with rest
- Depression, anxiety, or mood instability
- Brain fog and difficulty concentrating
- Frequent infections or slow wound healing
- Sensitivity to chemicals and medications
- High homocysteine levels on blood tests
- Difficulty detoxifying alcohol or medications
- Pregnancy complications or fertility issues

Lisa's Journey: Lisa had struggled with depression and chronic fatigue for years. Multiple doctors couldn't find anything wrong until genetic testing revealed she had two copies of the C677T variant. With targeted nutritional support for her methylation system, her energy returned and her mood stabilized. "I finally understood why standard treatments weren't working for me," she said.

MTHFR-Specific Anti-Inflammatory Nutrition

Key Nutrients for MTHFR Variants:

- ❖ Methylfolate (Not Folic Acid):
- MTHFR variants can't efficiently convert synthetic folic acid to the active form
- Food sources: Dark leafy greens, asparagus, Brussels sprouts, lentils
- Supplement form: 5-methyltetrahydrofolate (5-MTHF)
- Dosage: Typically 400-800 mcg daily, but individualized based on variants

- ❖ Active B12 (Methylcobalamin):
- Works synergistically with methylfolate
- Food sources: Wild-caught fish, grass-fed meat, nutritional yeast
- Supplement form: Methylcobalamin or adenosylcobalamin
- Avoid cyanocobalamin, which requires methylation to activate

- ❖ B6 (P5P):
- The active form is pyridoxal-5-phosphate (P5P)
- Food sources: Wild-caught salmon, chicken, sweet potatoes, sunflower seeds
- Important for neurotransmitter production and inflammation control

- ❖ Riboflavin (B2):
- Essential for MTHFR enzyme function
- Food sources: Almonds, mushrooms, eggs, leafy greens
- Many people with MTHFR variants need higher amounts

- ❖ Betaine (Trimethylglycine):
- Provides an alternative methylation pathway
- Food sources: Beets, spinach, quinoa, sweet potatoes
- Can be particularly helpful for those with severe MTHFR impairments

Foods That Support vs. Hinder Methylation

- ❖ Methylation-Supporting Foods:
- Cruciferous Vegetables: Broccoli, cabbage, kale provide compounds that support detoxification
- Sulfur-Rich Foods: Garlic, onions, eggs support glutathione production
- Beets: Rich in betaine, a natural methyl donor
- Organ Meats: Liver is particularly rich in B vitamins (if you can tolerate it)
- Sea Vegetables: Provide minerals needed for enzyme function

- ❖ Foods That Hinder Methylation:
- Fortified Foods with Folic Acid: Can block folate receptors in MTHFR variants
- Processed Foods: High in synthetic vitamins and low in cofactors
- Excess Alcohol: Depletes B vitamins and impairs methylation
- High-Sugar Foods: Increase inflammatory burden and deplete nutrients

Lifestyle Factors for MTHFR Variants

- ❖ Reduce Methylation Burden:
- Minimize exposure to toxins that require methylation for detoxification
- Support liver function with milk thistle, NAC, or other liver-supporting compounds
- Manage stress, as chronic stress depletes methylation resources
- Avoid medications that interfere with folate metabolism when possible

- ❖ Support Methylation Function:
- Regular moderate exercise supports methylation
- Adequate sleep allows for cellular repair processes
- Sauna or other heat therapy can support detoxification
- Mindfulness practices help manage stress and support neurotransmitter balance

FTO GENE: THE "FAT GENE" THAT'S REALLY ABOUT MUCH MORE

The FTO (Fat mass and Obesity-associated) gene is often called the "obesity gene," but this oversimplifies its role. FTO variants affect:
- How your body responds to different types of dietary fats
- Your appetite regulation and satiety signals
- Your metabolic response to exercise
- Your inflammatory response to certain foods
- Your circadian rhythm regulation

FTO Variants and Personalized Nutrition

- ❖ Common FTO Variants:
- AA genotype (about 16% of people): Higher sensitivity to dietary fats and calories
- AT genotype (about 48% of people): Moderate sensitivity
- TT genotype (about 36% of people): Lower sensitivity, better fat metabolism

Dietary Strategies Based on FTO Status

For FTO AA Carriers (Higher Sensitivity):

- ❖ Optimize Fat Quality and Quantity:
- Focus on anti-inflammatory fats: olive oil, avocados, nuts, seeds, and fatty fish
- Limit total fat intake to about 25-30% of calories
- Avoid saturated and trans fats, which may be more inflammatory for AA carriers
- Time fat intake earlier in the day when metabolism is higher

- ❖ Enhance Satiety:
- Emphasize protein and fiber to improve satiety signals
- Include foods that naturally suppress appetite: green tea, grapefruit, and protein-rich foods
- Eat slowly and mindfully to allow satiety hormones to function properly

- ❖ Support Metabolic Function:
- Regular physical activity is particularly important for AA carriers
- Strength training helps improve insulin sensitivity
- High-intensity interval training may be especially beneficial

Jennifer's Discovery: Jennifer had always struggled with weight despite eating what seemed like a healthy diet. Genetic testing revealed she was an FTO AA carrier. When she reduced her fat intake to 25% of calories (focusing on high-quality fats) and increased her protein and fiber, she finally achieved sustainable weight loss and reduced inflammation markers.

For FTO TT Carriers (Lower Sensitivity):

- ❖ Can Handle Higher Fat Intake:
- May thrive on up to 35-40% of calories from healthy fats
- Better tolerance for saturated fats from whole food sources
- May benefit from ketogenic or low-carb approaches
- Less likely to gain weight from dietary fat

- ❖ Different Exercise Response:
- May see better results from longer, moderate-intensity exercise
- Strength training remains important but may not need as high intensity
- May have better exercise recovery and adaptation

FTO and Inflammatory Response

- ❖ The Connection: FTO variants influence how your body responds to inflammatory triggers from food. This affects:
- Adipose Tissue Inflammation: AA carriers may develop more inflammatory fat tissue
- Insulin Sensitivity: FTO variants affect how well insulin works
- Cytokine Production: Different variants produce different inflammatory signals
- Recovery from Exercise: FTO affects how quickly you recover from inflammatory exercise stress

Personalized Anti-Inflammatory Strategies:

- ❖ For Higher-Risk FTO Variants (AA):

- More aggressive anti-inflammatory dietary approach needed
- Focus on omega-3 fatty acids and polyphenol-rich foods
- May need higher antioxidant intake
- Stress management particularly important
- Regular monitoring of inflammatory markers recommended

❖ For Lower-Risk FTO Variants (TT):
- More dietary flexibility while maintaining anti-inflammatory focus
- May tolerate occasional inflammatory foods better
- Still benefit from anti-inflammatory lifestyle but with less rigid requirements

PERSONALIZED POLYPHENOL SELECTION: YOUR GENETIC GUIDE TO SUPERFOODS

Polyphenols are powerful plant compounds that provide anti-inflammatory, antioxidant, and anti-aging benefits. However, your ability to absorb, metabolize, and benefit from different polyphenols depends significantly on your genetic makeup.

Key Genes Affecting Polyphenol Metabolism

❖ CYP1A2 (Caffeine Metabolism):
- Fast metabolizers (AA): Can handle more caffeine and may benefit from higher green tea intake
- Slow metabolizers (AC or CC): Should limit caffeine but may get more antioxidant benefits from lower amounts

❖ COMT (Dopamine Metabolism):
- Affects how you respond to certain polyphenols that influence neurotransmitters
- Met/Met: May be more sensitive to polyphenols that affect dopamine
- Val/Val: May need higher amounts of certain polyphenols for the same effect

❖ GSTP1 (Detoxification):
- Influences how well you handle certain polyphenols and their metabolites
- Affects optimal dosing of compounds like curcumin and resveratrol

Personalized Polyphenol Recommendations

❖ For Fast CYP1A2 Metabolizers:
- Green Tea: 3-4 cups daily may provide optimal benefits
- Coffee: Can handle 2-3 cups daily and may see cardiovascular benefits
- Dark Chocolate: Higher amounts (1-2 oz dark chocolate daily) may be beneficial
- Timing: Can consume caffeine-containing polyphenols later in the day

❖ For Slow CYP1A2 Metabolizers:
- Green Tea: 1-2 cups daily, focus on decaffeinated versions
- Coffee: Limit to 1 cup daily or switch to decaf
- White Tea: Lower caffeine alternative with similar polyphenols
- Timing: Consume caffeinated sources only in the morning

❖ For COMT Met/Met Carriers:
- Quercetin: Found in onions, apples, berries—may be particularly beneficial
- EGCG: From green tea, may have enhanced effects
- Resveratrol: From red grapes, may need lower doses
- Curcumin: May be more sensitive to mood and cognitive effects

- ❖ For COMT Val/Val Carriers:
- Higher Doses May Be Needed: Of most polyphenols for optimal effect
- Combination Therapy: May benefit from multiple polyphenol sources
- Consistency Important: Regular daily intake more important than high single doses

Food Sources for Personalized Polyphenol Intake

- ❖ High EGCG (Green Tea Polyphenols):
- Green tea (varies by processing and brewing)
- White tea (lower caffeine option)
- Matcha (concentrated form)

- ❖ Anthocyanins:
- Blueberries, blackberries, cherries
- Red and purple grapes
- Purple sweet potatoes
- Red cabbage

- ❖ Quercetin:
- Onions (particularly red onions)
- Apples (with skin)
- Berries
- Capers
- Red wine (in moderation)

- ❖ Curcumin:
- Turmeric (fresh or dried)
- Always combine with black pepper for absorption
- Fat-soluble, so consume with healthy fats

- ❖ Resveratrol:
- Red grapes and red wine
- Peanuts
- Dark berries
- Japanese knotweed (supplement source)

PHARMACOGENOMICS: HOW YOUR GENES AFFECT NATURAL COMPOUNDS

Just as people respond differently to pharmaceutical medications based on their genetics, they also respond differently to natural anti-inflammatory compounds. This field, called pharmacogenomics, helps explain why some people get amazing results from certain supplements while others see no benefit.

Key Genetic Factors Affecting Natural Compounds

- ❖ Phase I Detoxification (CYP Enzymes):
- CYP2D6: Affects metabolism of certain plant compounds
- CYP3A4: Influences how you process many herbal compounds
- CYP1A1: Affects polyphenol metabolism

- ❖ Phase II Detoxification:

- GSTT1 and GSTM1: Affect how you handle certain antioxidants
- UGT enzymes: Influence how you process and eliminate compounds
- SULT enzymes: Affect sulfur-containing compounds like those in cruciferous vegetables

❖ Transport Proteins:
- ABCB1: Affects how well certain compounds cross cell membranes
- SLCO1B1: Influences uptake of various natural compounds

Personalized Natural Anti-Inflammatory Protocols

❖ For Enhanced Detoxifiers:
- May need higher doses of natural compounds
- Can handle more aggressive detoxification protocols
- May benefit from cycling different compounds
- Can typically tolerate higher polyphenol intakes

❖ For Poor Detoxifiers:
- Start with lower doses and increase gradually
- Focus on supporting detoxification pathways first
- May be more sensitive to both benefits and side effects
- Need to be more careful with supplement combinations

❖ For Slow Metabolizers:
- Lower doses may be more effective
- Need longer time to see results
- May accumulate compounds, requiring dose adjustments
- Should space out different supplements throughout the day

Practical Implementation Guidelines

Getting Started Without Genetic Testing: While genetic testing provides the most precise information, you can still personalize your approach by:

1. Start Low and Go Slow: Begin with smaller amounts of any new compound and increase gradually
2. Track Your Response: Keep a detailed log of what you take and how you feel
3. Pay Attention to Sensitivity Signs: Headaches, digestive upset, or changes in sleep may indicate you need to adjust dosing
4. Work with Practitioners: Find healthcare providers familiar with nutrigenomics

❖ When to Consider Genetic Testing:
- You've tried multiple approaches with limited success
- You're sensitive to many foods or supplements
- You have a family history of certain conditions
- You want to optimize prevention strategies
- You're working with complex health conditions

Sample Personalized Protocols

❖ High Inflammation, Fast Metabolizer Protocol:
- Curcumin: 1000mg twice daily with black pepper and fat

- Omega-3s: 2-3g EPA/DHA daily
- Green tea extract: 400mg EGCG daily
- Quercetin: 500mg twice daily
- Resveratrol: 250mg daily

❖ Sensitive Individual, Slow Metabolizer Protocol:
- Curcumin: 250mg daily with meals
- Omega-3s: 1g EPA/DHA daily
- Green tea: 1-2 cups daily (or decaf extract)
- Quercetin: 250mg daily
- Focus on food sources of polyphenols rather than concentrated supplements

Putting It All Together: Your Personalized Action Plan

Step 1: Assess Your Current Genetic Knowledge

❖ What You Might Already Know:
- Family health history patterns
- How you respond to different foods
- Your sensitivity to caffeine and other compounds
- Previous genetic testing results (23andMe, AncestryDNA, etc.)

❖ What Additional Testing Might Help:
- Comprehensive nutrigenomics panels
- MTHFR testing specifically
- APOE status if you have cognitive concerns
- Functional medicine testing for methylation status

Step 2: Identify Your Priority Areas

Based on your health concerns and family history, prioritize which genetic factors are most relevant:
- Cognitive health: Focus on APOE status and related protocols
- Mood and energy: Emphasize MTHFR and methylation support
- Weight management: Consider FTO variants and personalized fat intake
- General inflammation: Look at polyphenol metabolism and detoxification capacity

Step 3: Implement Gradual Changes

Week 1-2: Basic anti-inflammatory foods for your suspected genetic profile
Week 3-4: Add targeted nutrients based on likely genetic variants
Week 5-8: Fine-tune based on your response and any new genetic information
Month 2+: Optimize and personalize further based on results

Step 4: Monitor and Adjust

❖ Subjective Measures:
- Energy levels throughout the day
- Mood stability and mental clarity
- Digestive comfort and regularity
- Sleep quality and recovery

- Exercise performance and recovery

❖ Objective Measures:
- Inflammatory markers (CRP, ESR)
- Homocysteine levels (for MTHFR variants)
- Lipid profiles (especially for APOE4 carriers)
- HbA1c and glucose control
- Body composition changes

Staying Ahead of the Curve

❖ What You Can Do Now:
- Stay informed about new research in nutrigenomics
- Consider genetic testing if it fits your budget and goals
- Work with practitioners who understand personalized medicine
- Track your responses to different interventions systematically
- Join communities focused on personalized health approaches

Remember the Key Principles

1. Your Genes Are Not Your Destiny: They're instructions, not commands
2. Knowledge Is Power: Understanding your genetic variants empowers better choices
3. Personalization Beats Generalization: What works for others may not work for you, and that's okay
4. Small Changes, Big Results: Targeted interventions based on genetics can be very effective
5. Evolution, Not Revolution: Gradual, sustainable changes work better than dramatic overhauls

Your genetics load the gun, but your lifestyle pulls the trigger. Understanding both gives you the power to choose your health destiny.

Chapter 3 Key Takeaways

❖ What You Learned:
- Your genetic variants influence how you respond to different foods and compounds, but they don't determine your health destiny
- APOE4 carriers need specific anti-inflammatory strategies focusing on lower saturated fat and higher omega-3 intake
- MTHFR variants require active forms of B vitamins and methylation support for optimal inflammation control
- FTO variants affect how your body responds to dietary fats and may influence your optimal macronutrient ratios
- Polyphenol metabolism varies by genetics, affecting which "superfoods" work best for you
- Natural compounds affect people differently based on their genetic detoxification and transport systems

❖ What You Can Do Right Now:
- Reflect on your family health history and your personal responses to different foods and compounds
- If you have existing genetic data, look up your variants for APOE, MTHFR, FTO, and CYP1A2
- Start implementing dietary strategies based on your most likely genetic profile
- Begin tracking your responses to different anti-inflammatory foods and compounds
- Consider working with a practitioner trained in nutrigenomics for personalized guidance

Chapter 4

Metabolic Flexibility and Inflammatory Adaptation

Your body is like a hybrid car that can run on different fuels. When you teach it to switch between these fuels efficiently, inflammation naturally decreases and energy naturally increases.

Imagine you had a car that could only run on premium gasoline, but you lived in a world where premium gas was only available a few hours each day. The rest of the time, your car would sputter, struggle, or break down completely. This is exactly what's happening in your body when you lose metabolic flexibility.

Your body was designed to be a metabolic masterpiece—capable of smoothly switching between different fuel sources depending on what's available and what you need. But modern eating patterns have locked most people into using only one fuel efficiently, creating a cascade of inflammatory problems that affect every aspect of your health.

UNDERSTANDING YOUR BODY'S FUEL SYSTEMS

Your Metabolic Engine: Built for Versatility

Think of your body as having two primary fuel systems, like a sophisticated hybrid vehicle:

- ❖ System 1: The Sugar Burner (Glucose Metabolism)
- Quick, readily available energy
- Burns fast and hot
- Provides immediate fuel for high-intensity activities
- Dominant system in most modern people

- ❖ System 2: The Fat Burner (Fat/Ketone Metabolism)
- Slow, steady, long-lasting energy
- Burns clean with minimal inflammatory byproducts
- Provides sustained fuel for endurance and mental clarity
- Underutilized system in most modern people

The Problem: Most people today are stuck in sugar-burning mode 24/7. It's like driving a hybrid car that never switches to electric mode—you're missing out on the efficiency, power, and reduced emissions that come from using all your available systems.

The Inflammatory Consequences of Metabolic Inflexibility

When you can only burn sugar efficiently, several inflammatory problems develop:

- Constant Hunger and Cravings: Your body runs out of easily accessible fuel every few hours, triggering stress hormones and inflammatory hunger signals.

- Blood Sugar Roller Coaster: Repeated spikes and crashes in blood sugar create inflammatory oxidative stress throughout your body.

- Fat Storage Mode: Excess sugar gets stored as fat, particularly inflammatory belly fat that actively produces inflammatory chemicals.

- Energy Crashes: Without access to your fat-burning system, you experience the 3 PM energy crash, morning fatigue, and exercise exhaustion.

Mike's Metabolic Awakening: Mike, a 42-year-old teacher, was eating every 2-3 hours to avoid energy crashes. He'd wake up hungry, get shaky if he missed a meal, and could barely function without his afternoon snack. When he learned to activate his fat-burning system, he could easily go 12-16 hours feeling energetic and clear-headed. "I didn't realize how much my constant eating was actually making me more tired," he said.

THE ANTI-INFLAMMATORY POWER OF KETONES

Ketones are special molecules your body produces when it burns fat efficiently. Think of them as premium fuel that burns cleaner, lasts longer, and produces fewer inflammatory byproducts than sugar.

What Are Ketones?
When your body breaks down fat for fuel, your liver converts fatty acids into ketone bodies. These molecules can cross into your brain, muscles, and other organs, providing efficient, clean-burning energy.

The Ketone Anti-Inflammatory Advantage

Ketones are like having a built-in anti-inflammatory medicine cabinet:

- Direct Anti-Inflammatory Signaling: Ketones don't just provide energy—they actively signal your body to reduce inflammation. The main ketone, beta-hydroxybutyrate, directly inhibits inflammatory pathways while activating healing ones.

- Antioxidant Production: Ketone metabolism increases production of your body's most powerful antioxidants, including glutathione, which protects your cells from inflammatory damage.

- Cellular Cleanup: Ketones promote autophagy—your body's natural process of cleaning out damaged cellular components that would otherwise trigger inflammation.

- Brain Protection: Ketones provide superior fuel for your brain while protecting neurons from inflammatory damage. This is why many people experience improved mental clarity when they become metabolically flexible.

- Mitochondrial Health: Ketones support the health of your cellular powerhouses (mitochondria), leading to more efficient energy production with less inflammatory waste.

Amber's Cognitive Transformation: Amber, a 38-year-old accountant, struggled with afternoon brain fog that made complex tasks nearly impossible. When she learned to tap into ketone production through metabolic flexibility training, her mental clarity improved dramatically. "It was like someone turned on the lights in my brain," she described. "I could think clearly all day long for the first time in years."

The Metabolic Flexibility Sweet Spot

The goal isn't to be in ketosis all the time—it's to be able to smoothly switch between fuel systems as needed. This flexibility provides:
- Stable energy throughout the day
- Reduced inflammation from both fuel systems
- Optimal performance for different activities
- Freedom from constant eating and food obsession
- Enhanced stress resilience and recovery

METABOLIC SWITCHING PROTOCOLS FOR INFLAMMATORY HEALING

Developing metabolic flexibility isn't about jumping into extreme measures—it's about gradually training your body to efficiently use both fuel systems. Think of it like training for a marathon: you start slowly and build endurance over time.

Phase 1: Foundation Building (Weeks 1-2)

Goal: Stabilize blood sugar and reduce inflammatory food reactions

- ❖ Morning Protocol:
- Start your day with protein and healthy fats instead of carbohydrates
- Examples: Eggs with avocado, Greek yogurt with nuts, or a protein smoothie with spinach
- This prevents the morning blood sugar spike that can trigger inflammation all day

- ❖ Meal Timing:
- Eat three balanced meals without snacking
- Allow 4-5 hours between meals
- This gives your body time to start accessing stored fat between meals

- ❖ Evening Protocol:
- Stop eating 3 hours before bedtime
- This allows your body to begin overnight fat burning and cellular repair processes

Real Example: Jennifer started by simply eating eggs and avocado for breakfast instead of her usual cereal and banana. Within three days, she noticed she wasn't crashing by 10 AM and could easily make it to lunch without snacking. "Such a simple change, but it made my whole morning different," she noted.

Phase 2: Flexibility Training (Weeks 3-6)

Goal: Teach your body to switch between fuel systems efficiently

- ❖ 12-Hour Eating Window:
- Eat all meals within a 12-hour period (e.g., 7 AM to 7 PM)
- This creates a natural 12-hour fasting period for fat burning practice
- Start with whatever feels comfortable and gradually extend

- ❖ Strategic Carbohydrate Timing:
- Eat most carbohydrates around physical activity when your body can use them immediately
- Focus on nutrient-dense carbs like sweet potatoes, berries, and vegetables
- Avoid refined carbs that cause inflammatory blood sugar spikes

❖ Movement Integration:
- Take walks after meals to help clear glucose from your bloodstream
- Try gentle exercise in a fasted state to encourage fat burning
- Listen to your body and adjust intensity based on how you feel

Phase 3: Advanced Flexibility (Weeks 7+)

Goal: Achieve smooth metabolic switching with maximum anti-inflammatory benefits

❖ Extended Eating Windows:
- Gradually work toward 14-16 hour eating windows if comfortable
- Some people naturally settle into eating 2-3 meals per day
- The goal is what feels sustainable and energizing for you

❖ Activity-Based Fueling:
- Use your body's signals to determine when and what to eat
- High-intensity activities may require strategic carbohydrate timing
- Low-intensity, longer activities can often be fueled by fat stores

❖ Stress and Sleep Integration:
- Adjust your eating patterns based on stress levels and sleep quality
- High stress or poor sleep may require more frequent meals temporarily
- Use metabolic flexibility as a tool, not a rigid rule

Troubleshooting Common Challenges

❖ "I Feel Tired and Cranky":
This is normal during the first 1-2 weeks as your body adapts. Support yourself with:
- Extra sleep and stress management
- Adequate salt and electrolytes
- Gradual rather than dramatic changes
- Patience with the adaptation process

❖ "I Can't Stop Thinking About Food":
Food obsession often indicates:
- Inadequate nutrition in your meals
- Emotional or stress eating patterns
- Too rapid progression in fasting periods
- Need for professional support with eating behaviors

❖ "My Workouts Suffer":
Athletic performance may temporarily decrease as your body adapts:
- Reduce workout intensity during the first 2-3 weeks
- Consider strategic carbohydrate timing around workouts
- Focus on fat adaptation before worrying about performance
- Remember that adaptation takes time but results in better long-term performance

HOW DIFFERENT FOODS AFFECT YOUR INFLAMMATORY RESPONSE

Every time you eat, your body mounts what's called a postprandial (after-meal) inflammatory response. This is normal and healthy when it's brief and controlled. Problems arise when this response is excessive or prolonged.

Macronutrient Inflammatory Profiles

❖ High-Carbohydrate Meals:
- Cause rapid blood sugar and insulin spikes
- Trigger inflammatory oxidative stress
- Activate inflammatory pathways for 2-4 hours after eating
- Create a cycle of hunger and cravings within 2-3 hours

The Breakfast Experiment: Tom tested his blood sugar response to different breakfasts using a continuous glucose monitor. His usual bagel and orange juice caused his blood sugar to spike to 180 mg/dL and stay elevated for over 3 hours. The same morning, his wife ate eggs, avocado, and berries—her blood sugar barely moved above 100 mg/dL. "Seeing the actual numbers was mind-blowing," Tom said. "I had no idea how much that bagel was stressing my system."

❖ High-Fat Meals:
- Provide steady, sustained energy release
- Minimal impact on blood sugar and insulin
- Support anti-inflammatory signaling pathways
- Promote satiety for 4-6 hours or more

❖ Protein-Rich Meals:
- Moderate, controlled impact on blood sugar
- Support muscle maintenance and metabolism
- Provide sustained satiety
- Require energy to digest, boosting metabolism

❖ Balanced Meals (Optimal Approach):
- Combine all macronutrients in anti-inflammatory ratios
- Moderate blood sugar response
- Sustained energy and satiety
- Support metabolic flexibility development

The Inflammatory Food Timing Strategy

*Morning: Start with protein and fat to stabilize blood sugar for the entire day
*Mid-Day: Include moderate amounts of nutrient-dense carbohydrates when you're most active
*Evening: Focus on protein and vegetables to support overnight recovery and fat burning

Meal Composition for Metabolic Flexibility

❖ The Anti-Inflammatory Plate:
- 1/2 plate: Non-starchy vegetables (anti-inflammatory compounds and fiber)
- 1/4 plate: High-quality protein (metabolic support and satiety)
- 1/4 plate: Healthy fats and/or nutrient-dense carbohydrates (sustained energy)

❖ Specific Food Combinations That Reduce Inflammation:
- Salmon with roasted vegetables and avocado
- Grass-fed beef with sweet potato and sauerkraut

- Eggs with spinach, mushrooms, and olive oil
- Chicken with broccoli and coconut oil
- Sardines with mixed greens and nuts

EXERCISE: YOUR METABOLIC FLEXIBILITY ACCELERATOR

Exercise isn't just about burning calories—it's about training your body to efficiently switch between fuel systems while building inflammatory resilience.

The Anti-Inflammatory Exercise Prescription

- ❖ Low-Intensity, Fat-Burning Activities (60-70% of training time):
- Walking, especially after meals
- Easy swimming or cycling
- Yoga or tai chi
- Recreational hiking
- Light resistance training

These activities:
- Train your fat-burning system
- Reduce inflammatory stress
- Can be done daily without overtraining
- Provide sustainable, long-term benefits

- ❖ Moderate-Intensity, Metabolic Training (20-30% of training time):
- Brisk walking or jogging
- Circuit training
- Dancing
- Sports activities
- Moderate resistance training

These activities:
- Improve cardiovascular health
- Build metabolic flexibility
- Enhance insulin sensitivity
- Provide mood and energy benefits

- ❖ High-Intensity, Performance Training (5-10% of training time):
- Sprint intervals
- Heavy resistance training
- High-intensity sports
- Challenging athletic pursuits

These activities:
- Build power and performance
- Stimulate adaptive responses
- Require adequate recovery
- Should be used strategically, not constantly

The Metabolic Flexibility Workout Plan

- ❖ Week 1-2: Foundation Phase
- Daily 20-30 minute walks
- 2-3 gentle yoga or stretching sessions
- 1-2 light resistance training sessions
- Focus on consistency over intensity

- ❖ Week 3-6: Building Phase
- Daily movement (walking, yoga, or light activity)
- 2-3 moderate-intensity training sessions
- 1 higher-intensity session per week
- Include one completely restful day

- ❖ Week 7+: Maintenance Phase
- Intuitive movement based on energy levels
- Mix of intensities throughout the week
- Regular assessment and adjustment
- Focus on sustainable, enjoyable activities

Exercise Timing for Maximum Anti-Inflammatory Benefits

- ❖ Morning Movement:
- Gentle activity in a fasted state promotes fat burning
- Helps establish circadian rhythms
- Sets positive tone for the entire day
- Can be as simple as 10-15 minutes of walking or stretching

- ❖ Post-Meal Movement:
- Even 2-3 minutes of walking after meals improves blood sugar control
- Reduces post-meal inflammatory responses
- Aids digestion and prevents energy crashes
- Easy to incorporate into daily routines

- ❖ Evening Movement:
- Gentle, restorative activities promote better sleep
- Helps process daily stress and tension
- Avoid high-intensity exercise close to bedtime
- Focus on relaxation and recovery

Vanessa's Discovery: Vanessa, a busy marketing director, thought she needed intense hour-long workouts to see results. When she switched to 15-minute morning walks, 2-minute post-meal movement breaks, and 20-minute evening yoga sessions, she lost more weight, had better energy, and felt less stressed than with her previous intense workout regimen. "Less was definitely more in my case," she realized.

ACTIVATING YOUR BODY'S METABOLIC FURNACE: BROWN FAT

The Fat That Burns Fat

Not all fat in your body is the same. You have two main types:
- White fat: Stores energy and can produce inflammatory chemicals when excessive
- Brown fat: Burns energy to produce heat and has powerful anti-inflammatory properties

Brown adipose tissue (BAT) is like having a metabolic furnace that burns calories while producing anti-inflammatory compounds. The more active your brown fat, the better your metabolic flexibility and inflammatory control.

The Brown Fat Advantage

- ❖ Metabolic Benefits:
- Burns calories 24/7, even at rest
- Improves insulin sensitivity
- Enhances overall metabolic rate
- Supports weight management without dieting

- ❖ Anti-Inflammatory Benefits:
- Produces anti-inflammatory molecules
- Reduces systemic inflammation
- Protects against metabolic diseases
- Supports healthy aging processes

How to Activate Your Brown Fat

- ❖ Cold Exposure (The Most Powerful Method):
- End showers with 30-60 seconds of cold water
- Spend time outdoors in cool weather
- Keep your home slightly cooler (65-68°F)
- Try ice baths or cold plunges if available

Start Slowly: Begin with 15-30 seconds of cold water at the end of your shower. Gradually increase the duration as your body adapts. The goal is mild discomfort, not misery.

- ❖ Exercise Activation:
- Regular physical activity stimulates brown fat
- High-intensity intervals are particularly effective
- Resistance training also promotes brown fat activity
- Consistency matters more than intensity

- ❖ Dietary Support:
- Green tea contains compounds that activate brown fat
- Capsaicin from chili peppers stimulates brown fat
- Menthol from mint can trigger brown fat activation
- Avoid overeating, which can suppress brown fat activity

- ❖ Sleep and Stress Management:
- Quality sleep supports brown fat function
- Chronic stress suppresses brown fat activity
- Meditation and relaxation techniques help
- Consistent sleep schedules optimize brown fat activation

The Brown Fat Lifestyle Protocol

- ❖ Morning:
- Wake up in a cool room (around 65°F)

- End your shower with 30-60 seconds of cold water
- Have green tea with breakfast
- Get outside for morning light and fresh air

- ❖ Throughout the Day:
- Keep your workspace slightly cool
- Take breaks outside, especially in cooler weather
- Stay hydrated with cool (not ice-cold) water
- Avoid overheating with excessive layers

- ❖ Evening:
- Lower your home temperature for sleeping
- Avoid large meals close to bedtime
- Practice stress-reduction techniques
- Ensure adequate sleep duration and quality

Michael's Brown Fat Experiment: Michael, a 45-year-old accountant, was skeptical about cold exposure until he tried it consistently for 30 days. He started with 20-second cold shower endings and gradually worked up to 60 seconds. Within a month, he noticed improved energy, better sleep, enhanced mood, and easier weight management. "I never thought something so simple could make such a big difference," he said.

Your Metabolic Flexibility Assessment

Before starting your metabolic flexibility journey, it's helpful to understand your current state. Rate yourself on the following indicators (1 = never, 5 = always):

- ❖ Energy Stability:
- I can go 4-5 hours between meals without getting hungry or irritable (___/5)
- My energy levels are stable throughout the day (___/5)
- I don't experience afternoon energy crashes (___/5)
- I wake up feeling refreshed and energized (___/5)

- ❖ Food Flexibility:
- I can skip a meal occasionally without feeling awful (___/5)
- I don't obsess about food or meal timing (___/5)
- I can eat different types of meals without digestive distress (___/5)
- I don't get shaky or anxious when hungry (___/5)

- ❖ Exercise Performance:
- I can exercise comfortably without needing to eat immediately before (___/5)
- My workout performance is consistent regardless of meal timing (___/5)
- I recover quickly from physical activity (___/5)
- I enjoy both high and low-intensity activities (___/5)

- ❖ Metabolic Markers:
- I maintain stable weight without obsessive food monitoring (___/5)
- I don't experience intense cravings for specific foods (___/5)
- My sleep quality is good and consistent (___/5)
- I handle stress well without turning to food (___/5)

Total Score: ___/80

❖ Interpreting Your Results:
- 60-80: Excellent metabolic flexibility
- 45-59: Good flexibility with room for improvement
- 30-44: Moderate flexibility—targeted improvements will help significantly
- Below 30: Poor flexibility—systematic approach recommended

Your 30-Day Metabolic Flexibility Transformation Plan

❖ Week 1: Foundation
Daily Goals:
- Eat protein and fat for breakfast
- Allow 4-5 hours between meals
- End showers with 30 seconds of cold water
- Take a 10-minute walk after dinner

Weekly Goals:
- Plan and prepare 3 metabolically balanced meals
- Try 2 new anti-inflammatory recipes
- Get 7-8 hours of sleep nightly
- Complete 2 gentle exercise sessions

❖ Week 2: Building
Daily Goals:
- Maintain 12-hour eating window
- Include movement after each meal
- Practice one stress-reduction technique
- Keep home temperature at 65-68°F

Weekly Goals:
- Increase cold shower duration to 45 seconds
- Add 1 moderate-intensity exercise session
- Try eating 2 meals instead of 3 on one day
- Track energy levels and mood daily

❖ Week 3: Expanding
Daily Goals:
- Extend eating window to 14 hours if comfortable
- Include fat-burning exercise 4 days
- Practice mindful eating at each meal
- Get morning sunlight exposure

Weekly Goals:
- Try 60-second cold showers
- Add 1 higher-intensity exercise session
- Experiment with different meal compositions
- Assess progress and adjust as needed

❖ Week 4: Integration
Daily Goals:
- Eat intuitively based on hunger and energy

- Move your body in ways that feel good
- Practice gratitude for your body's capabilities
- Maintain consistent sleep schedule

Weekly Goals:
- Create your personalized long-term plan
- Identify your most effective strategies
- Set realistic goals for continued progress
- Celebrate your improvements and insights

Common Challenges and Solutions

❖ "I Feel Cold All the Time":
This often indicates thyroid or metabolic issues:
- Start more gradually with changes
- Ensure adequate nutrition, especially protein
- Check with a healthcare provider about thyroid function
- Focus on gentle warming activities like movement

❖ "I'm Not Losing Weight":
Weight loss isn't the only marker of metabolic health:
- Focus on energy, mood, and sleep improvements
- Ensure you're eating enough to support metabolism
- Consider that muscle gain may offset fat loss
- Remember that sustainable changes take time

❖ "I Can't Stop Thinking About Food":
This suggests inadequate nutrition or emotional eating:
- Increase protein and fat intake
- Address underlying stress and emotions
- Consider working with a counselor or nutritionist
- Ensure you're eating enough overall calories

❖ "My Workouts Are Suffering":
Athletic performance may temporarily decrease:
- Reduce workout intensity during adaptation
- Ensure adequate fuel around training sessions
- Be patient—adaptation can take 2-6 weeks
- Consider working with a sports nutritionist

The Metabolic Flexibility Lifestyle

The goal isn't perfection—it's creating a sustainable lifestyle that supports your body's natural metabolic intelligence. This means:

- Flexibility Over Rigidity: Use these principles as guidelines, not absolute rules. Your body's needs may vary based on stress, activity levels, health status, and life circumstances.

- Progress Over Perfection: Small, consistent improvements matter more than dramatic changes that can't be maintained.

- Individual Adaptation: What works for others may not work exactly the same for you. Pay attention to your body's responses and adjust accordingly.

- Long-Term Perspective: Focus on how you feel and function rather than just external measures like weight or appearance.

Your Metabolic Flexibility Future

As you develop metabolic flexibility, you'll likely experience:
- Stable energy throughout the day
- Freedom from constant hunger and food obsession
- Better stress resilience and recovery
- Improved athletic performance over time
- Enhanced mental clarity and mood stability
- Reduced inflammation and chronic disease risk
- Greater confidence in your body's abilities

The Science Made Simple

- Metabolic Flexibility = Your body's ability to efficiently switch between different fuel sources based on availability and need.

- Ketones = Clean-burning fuel molecules produced when your body breaks down fat, providing energy while reducing inflammation.

- Brown Fat = Special fat tissue that burns calories to produce heat while creating anti-inflammatory compounds.

- Postprandial Response = Your body's reaction to eating, including blood sugar, insulin, and inflammatory changes.

- Metabolic Switching = The process of training your body to efficiently use both glucose and fat for fuel.

Metabolic flexibility isn't about restriction—it's about restoration. You're not forcing your body to do something unnatural; you're removing the obstacles that prevent it from doing what it was designed to do.

Chapter 4 Key Takeaways

❖ What You Learned:
- Metabolic flexibility—the ability to switch between fuel sources—is crucial for reducing inflammation
- Ketones provide clean-burning energy while actively reducing inflammatory pathways
- Different macronutrients create different inflammatory responses after meals
- Strategic exercise timing can enhance metabolic flexibility and inflammatory resilience
- Brown fat activation provides metabolic and anti-inflammatory benefits

❖ What You Can Do Right Now:
- Start your next meal with protein and healthy fats instead of carbohydrates
- Take a 2-3 minute walk after eating to help process the meal
- End your next shower with 15-30 seconds of cool water

- Assess your current metabolic flexibility using the chapter questionnaire
- Choose one protocol from the 30-day plan to implement this week

Chapter 5

Your Gut's Secret Control Center

Your gut bacteria aren't just passengers along for the ride—they're the drivers of your inflammatory response. Learning to work with them instead of against them could be the key to transforming your health.

Imagine if I told you that living inside your body right now are trillions of tiny organisms that have more control over your health than your own genes. You might think that sounds like science fiction, but it's science fact. These microscopic partners—your gut bacteria—are constantly communicating with your immune system, telling it when to turn inflammation on and when to turn it off.

Here's what might surprise you even more: you can actually influence these conversations. By understanding how your gut bacteria talk to your immune system, you can essentially reprogram your body's inflammatory responses. This isn't about taking random probiotics from the drugstore—it's about precision healing using specific bacterial strains that scientists have discovered can dramatically reduce inflammation.

Let me show you how this incredible system works and, more importantly, how you can use this knowledge to feel better than you have in years.

YOUR INTERNAL ECOSYSTEM: MORE THAN JUST DIGESTION

The Numbers Will Amaze You

Your gut contains:
- 38 trillion bacteria (that's more bacterial cells than human cells in your body)
- Over 1,000 different species of bacteria
- Genes from these bacteria that outnumber your human genes 100 to 1
- A communication network more complex than the internet

Think of your gut as a bustling city with different neighborhoods. Some neighborhoods are filled with helpful citizens (beneficial bacteria) who keep the peace, clean up waste, and contribute to the community. Other neighborhoods might harbor troublemakers (harmful bacteria) who create chaos and inflammation.

The health of your entire body depends on which type of citizens dominate your internal city.

Your Gut's Inflammation Control Center

Deep within your gut lining are special cells that act like security guards. Scientists call these the "inflammasome"—think of them as your body's internal fire department. These security guards are constantly receiving reports from your gut bacteria about what's happening in your digestive system.

Here's how the conversation works:

- Good Bacteria Report: "All quiet here. Food looks safe. No threats detected. Keep inflammation levels low."

- Bad Bacteria Report: "Emergency! Toxic substances detected! Barrier compromised! Sound the alarm! Increase inflammation now!"

Your inflammasome listens to these reports and adjusts your body's inflammatory response accordingly. The problem is, in our modern world, the bad bacteria often outnumber the good ones, so your inflammasome is getting constant emergency reports even when there's no real danger.

THE BACTERIAL STRAINS THAT CAN CHANGE YOUR LIFE

You've probably seen probiotic supplements in the store, but here's what most people don't know: different bacterial strains have completely different effects on your body. It's like the difference between different types of workers—you wouldn't hire a plumber to fix your car or an electrician to bake your wedding cake.

Let me introduce you to some specific bacterial strains that scientists have discovered can dramatically reduce inflammation:

The Anti-Inflammatory All-Stars

❖ Lactobacillus rhamnosus GG - The Gut Barrier Builder
- What it does: Strengthens your gut lining to prevent inflammatory toxins from entering your bloodstream
- Real-world impact: People with leaky gut syndrome often see dramatic improvements in bloating, food sensitivities, and energy levels
- Found in: Specific probiotic supplements and some fermented foods

❖ Bifidobacterium longum - The Mood Stabilizer
- What it does: Produces chemicals that directly communicate with your brain to reduce stress-induced inflammation
- Real-world impact: Studies show it can reduce anxiety and depression while lowering inflammatory markers
- Found in: Fermented dairy products and targeted probiotic supplements

❖ Lactobacillus casei Shirota - The Immune Educator
- What it does: Teaches your immune system to respond appropriately, reducing overactive inflammatory responses
- Real-world impact: Can help with allergies, autoimmune conditions, and frequent infections
- Found in: Specific fermented milk products and probiotic supplements

❖ Akkermansia muciniphila - The Metabolic Protector
- What it does: Maintains your gut lining and improves insulin sensitivity
- Real-world impact: Helps with weight management and reduces inflammation associated with diabetes
- Found in: Emerging in specialized probiotic supplements; can be increased through specific dietary approaches

Why Strain Specificity Matters

Think of bacterial strains like keys—each one is shaped differently and unlocks different biological processes. A strain that helps with digestive issues might not help with mood problems, and a strain that reduces allergy symptoms might not help with weight management.

This is why randomly taking generic probiotics often doesn't work. It's like having a ring of keys but not knowing which one opens which door.

THE SECRET CHEMICAL MESSENGERS: HOW BACTERIA TALK TO YOUR BODY

Your gut bacteria are like tiny chemical factories, constantly producing compounds that directly affect your health. Scientists call these compounds "postbiotics"—the beneficial chemicals that bacteria produce as they go about their daily lives.

Think of postbiotics as text messages between your bacteria and your body. These messages can tell your immune system to calm down, help repair damaged tissue, or even influence your mood and energy levels.

The Anti-Inflammatory Messengers

❖ Short-Chain Fatty Acids (SCFAs) - The Master Healers
These are probably the most important anti-inflammatory compounds your bacteria produce:

- Butyrate: Acts like fuel for your gut lining cells and directly turns off inflammatory pathways
- Propionate: Travels to your liver and helps regulate your immune system
- Acetate: Crosses into your brain and helps reduce neuroinflammation

How to increase them: Feed your bacteria the fiber they love from vegetables, fruits, and whole grains. Different types of fiber feed different bacteria, so variety is key.

❖ Gamma-Aminobutyric Acid (GABA) - The Natural Calm
Some bacteria produce this relaxing brain chemical directly in your gut:
- Reduces anxiety and stress-induced inflammation
- Helps with sleep quality
- Calms overactive immune responses

❖ Serotonin Precursors - The Mood Managers
About 90% of your body's serotonin is produced in your gut:
- Influences mood and emotional well-being
- Affects gut motility and digestion
- Impacts inflammation levels throughout your body

The Bacterial Pharmacy in Your Gut

Your gut bacteria are essentially running a personalized pharmacy, custom-making medications for your specific needs. The question is: are they making anti-inflammatory medicines or pro-inflammatory toxins?

The answer depends on what you feed them and how you treat them.

THE REVOLUTIONARY APPROACH: FECAL MICROBIOTA TRANSPLANTATION

Sometimes, the bacterial imbalance in your gut is so severe that adding probiotics is like trying to plant a garden in polluted soil. In these cases, doctors are now using a revolutionary approach called fecal microbiota transplantation (FMT).

How It Works

FMT involves taking healthy gut bacteria from a carefully screened donor and transplanting them into a patient's gut. Think of it as a "bacterial reset" that can rapidly restore a healthy gut ecosystem.

- ❖ The Process:
1. Donors are extensively screened for health and safety
2. The healthy microbiome is prepared in specialized labs
3. It's introduced into the patient's gut (usually through colonoscopy or capsules)
4. The new bacteria colonize and begin producing anti-inflammatory compounds

Remarkable Results for Inflammatory Conditions

- ❖ Inflammatory Bowel Disease (IBD):
- Some patients see complete remission of symptoms
- Inflammation markers drop dramatically
- Quality of life improves significantly

- ❖ Clostridioides difficile Infections:
- Success rates over 90% for recurrent infections
- Rapid restoration of gut health
- Prevention of life-threatening complications

The Future of FMT

Researchers are working on:
- Standardized bacterial cocktails that don't require individual donors
- Oral capsules that are easier to take than colonoscopy procedures
- Targeted treatments for specific inflammatory conditions
- Personalized bacterial formulations based on individual needs

Important Note: FMT is still a medical procedure that requires professional supervision. However, understanding how it works can help you appreciate the power of microbiome restoration and guide your own gut healing journey.

FEEDING YOUR ANTI-INFLAMMATORY ARMY: THE PREBIOTIC REVOLUTION

Probiotics are the beneficial bacteria, but prebiotics are the food that keeps them healthy and active. Think of prebiotics as fertilizer for your internal garden—without the right nutrients, even the best bacteria can't do their job.

The Fiber Pharmacy

Different types of fiber feed different bacteria, and each type of bacteria produces different anti-inflammatory compounds. This is why fiber diversity is so important:

- ❖ Inulin - Feeds Bifidobacteria
- Sources: Jerusalem artichokes, garlic, onions, leeks
- Benefits: Increases production of anti-inflammatory SCFAs
- Helps with: Digestive health, immune function, mineral absorption

- ❖ Beta-Glucan - Feeds Lactobacilli
- Sources: Oats, barley, mushrooms
- Benefits: Reduces inflammatory markers, supports immune function
- Helps with: Heart health, blood sugar control, cholesterol management

- ❖ Resistant Starch - Feeds Butyrate-Producing Bacteria
- Sources: Cooked and cooled potatoes, green bananas, legumes
- Benefits: Produces high levels of butyrate for gut healing
- Helps with: Gut barrier function, insulin sensitivity, colon health

- ❖ Pectin - Feeds Akkermansia
- Sources: Apples, citrus fruits, berries
- Benefits: Strengthens gut lining, reduces inflammation
- Helps with: Metabolic health, weight management, gut barrier integrity

The Prebiotic Combination Strategy

Research shows that combining different types of prebiotic fibers is more effective than using just one type. Think of it like feeding a diverse community—everyone has different nutritional needs.

- ❖ The Daily Fiber Rainbow:
- Red: Apples, berries (pectin)
- Orange: Sweet potatoes, carrots (various fibers)
- Yellow: Bananas, corn (resistant starch)
- Green: Leafy greens, broccoli (diverse fibers)
- Blue/Purple: Blueberries, purple cabbage (anthocyanins + fiber)
- White: Onions, garlic, leeks (inulin)

Tom's Transformation: Tom had been taking probiotics for months with minimal results. When he started focusing on prebiotic diversity—eating at least 5 different colored plant foods daily—his digestive issues improved dramatically within 2 weeks. "I realized I was starving my good bacteria," he said.

Prebiotic Supplements: When Food Isn't Enough

Sometimes, especially if you're dealing with significant gut damage, you may need concentrated prebiotic supplements:

- ❖ Galacto-oligosaccharides (GOS):
- Particularly effective for increasing Bifidobacteria
- Well-tolerated by most people
- Good for starting gut healing

- ❖ Fructo-oligosaccharides (FOS):
- Feeds multiple beneficial bacteria strains
- Start with small amounts to avoid digestive upset
- Combine with other prebiotics for best results

- ❖ Modified Citrus Pectin:
- Specifically supports Akkermansia growth
- Has additional detoxification benefits
- Good for people with metabolic issues

YOUR PERSONAL INFLAMMATION DASHBOARD: MICROBIOME TESTING

In the past, improving gut health was mostly guesswork. Now, advanced testing can show you exactly what's happening in your gut microbiome and guide precise interventions.

What Modern Testing Can Tell You

- ❖ Bacterial Diversity:
- How many different species you have (higher diversity = better health)
- Which beneficial bacteria are missing
- Which harmful bacteria are overgrown

- ❖ Inflammatory Markers:
- Calprotectin: Measures gut inflammation levels
- Secretory IgA: Shows immune system activity in your gut
- Zonulin: Indicates gut barrier integrity ("leaky gut")

- ❖ Functional Markers:
- SCFA production levels
- Digestive enzyme activity
- Bile acid metabolism

- ❖ Personalized Recommendations:
- Which specific probiotic strains you need
- Which prebiotic fibers would benefit you most
- Which foods might be triggering inflammation

Reading Your Results

Sample Report Translation:
"Low Akkermansia, elevated Enterobacteriaceae, reduced butyrate production"

- ❖ What this means in plain English:
- Your gut lining bacteria are depleted (Akkermansia)
- You have overgrowth of potentially inflammatory bacteria (Enterobacteriaceae)
- Your gut isn't producing enough healing compounds (butyrate)

- ❖ Action Plan:
- Increase pectin-rich foods (apples, berries) to feed Akkermansia
- Add specific anti-inflammatory probiotics
- Include more resistant starch to boost butyrate production
- Consider targeted antimicrobial herbs to reduce harmful bacteria

Lisa's Precision Approach: Lisa's test showed she had virtually no Bifidobacteria but high levels of inflammatory bacteria. Instead of random probiotics, she took a targeted Bifidobacterium supplement and increased her intake of foods that specifically fed these bacteria. Within 6 weeks, her chronic fatigue and brain fog resolved.

When to Test

❖ Consider testing if you have:
- Persistent digestive issues
- Chronic inflammation or autoimmune conditions
- Mood or cognitive problems
- Difficulty losing weight
- Frequent infections
- Poor response to standard probiotic supplements

❖ Follow-up testing:
- After 3-6 months of targeted interventions
- To track progress and adjust protocols
- Before and after major dietary changes

YOUR GUT-BRAIN-INFLAMMATION RESET

The 30-Day Challenge

Ready to experience the power of your microbiome? Here's a comprehensive 30-day protocol:

❖ Week 1: Foundation
- Eliminate processed foods, artificial sweeteners, and excess sugar
- Begin taking a broad-spectrum probiotic with at least 5 different strains
- Eat one fermented food daily (kefir, sauerkraut, kimchi, or miso)
- Include 3 different colored vegetables with each meal

❖ Week 2: Expansion
- Add resistant starch foods (cooked and cooled potatoes, green bananas)
- Increase total fiber intake gradually
- Include prebiotic-rich foods (garlic, onions, and Jerusalem artichokes)
- Start a stress-reduction practice (meditation, yoga, or deep breathing)

❖ Week 3: Diversification
- Aim for 25+ different plant foods for the week
- Try new fermented foods from different cultures
- Add targeted probiotics based on your specific symptoms
- Include gut-healing foods (bone broth, aloe vera, and slippery elm)

❖ Week 4: Optimization
- Fine-tune your protocol based on how you feel
- Continue expanding plant food diversity
- Add postbiotic supplements if needed
- Plan for long-term sustainability

Tracking Your Progress

❖ Daily Measurements:
- Energy levels (1-10 scale)
- Mood stability (1-10 scale)
- Digestive comfort (1-10 scale)
- Sleep quality (1-10 scale)

- ❖ Weekly Assessments:
- Overall inflammation symptoms
- Cognitive clarity and focus
- Exercise recovery
- Stress resilience

- ❖ Monthly Evaluations:
- Chronic symptom improvements
- Weight and body composition changes
- Laboratory markers (if testing)
- Quality of life measures

THE PARTNERSHIP APPROACH

Working with Your Microscopic Allies

The key to success is thinking of your gut bacteria as partners rather than passengers. They're not just along for the ride—they're actively working to keep you healthy when you provide the right environment.

- ❖ What Your Bacteria Need from You:
- Diverse, fiber-rich foods to eat
- Consistent feeding schedule
- Protection from harmful chemicals and medications
- Stress management to maintain a stable environment
- Adequate sleep for repair and maintenance

- ❖ What Your Bacteria Give You:
- Anti-inflammatory compounds that heal your body
- Neurotransmitters that stabilize your mood
- Immune system training that prevents overreactions
- Metabolic support for healthy weight and energy
- Protection against harmful pathogens

The Mutual Benefit System

This isn't a one-way relationship. When you take care of your gut bacteria, they take care of you. When you feed them well, they produce compounds that make you feel amazing. When you stress them with poor food choices or chronic stress, they produce inflammatory compounds that make you feel terrible.

Understanding this partnership changes everything about how you approach your health. Every meal becomes an opportunity to support your bacterial allies. Every lifestyle choice becomes a chance to strengthen this crucial relationship.

Your Microbiome-Powered Future

Imagine waking up each morning with stable energy that lasts all day. Picture your mind being clear and focused, your mood balanced and resilient. Envision your body free from chronic aches and pains, your digestion comfortable and efficient.

This isn't just wishful thinking—it's the power of a well-balanced, anti-inflammatory microbiome. The bacteria in your gut are capable of producing this transformation, but they need your partnership to make it happen.

The science is clear: your gut bacteria control your inflammation more than any other single factor. By working with them strategically, you can achieve health improvements that might seem impossible through other approaches.

Your journey to optimal health doesn't start in the gym or even in the kitchen—it starts in your gut, with the trillions of microscopic partners who are waiting to help you feel better than you ever thought possible.

Your gut bacteria are not just microbes—they're your personalized medicine manufacturers, working 24/7 to keep you healthy. The question isn't whether they're making medicine or poison—it's what kind of raw materials you're giving them to work with.

Chapter 5 Key Takeaways

- ❖ What You Learned:
- Your gut bacteria directly control your inflammatory responses through complex chemical communications
- Specific bacterial strains have specific anti-inflammatory effects—precision matters more than quantity
- Bacterial metabolites (postbiotics) are powerful anti-inflammatory compounds your body produces naturally
- Prebiotic fiber diversity is crucial for maintaining anti-inflammatory bacteria
- Modern testing can guide personalized microbiome interventions
- Your gut-brain connection means gut health directly affects mood, energy, and cognitive function

- ❖ What You Can Do Right Now:
- Start eating a wider variety of colorful plant foods to feed beneficial bacteria
- Choose fermented foods from different cultures to increase bacterial diversity
- If taking probiotics, research specific strains for your particular symptoms
- Track how different foods affect your energy, mood, and digestive comfort
- Consider comprehensive stool testing if you have chronic inflammatory symptoms

PART II

THE ANTI-INFLAMMATORY DIET FOUNDATION

Chapter 6

Core Principles of Anti-Inflammatory Eating

The best diet isn't about restriction—it's about nourishment. When you understand what your body truly needs, healthy choices become natural choices.

For decades, we've been taught that weight and health are simply about calories in versus calories out. But what if I told you that 200 calories of almonds affects your body completely differently than 200 calories of soda? What if the timing of when you eat matters as much as what you eat? What if your body has an internal clock that influences how it processes food?

This is where anti-inflammatory eating diverges from traditional dieting. Instead of focusing on restriction and deprivation, we focus on abundance—giving your body an abundance of the nutrients it needs to heal, thrive, and naturally regulate inflammation.

In this chapter, you'll discover the core principles that will guide every food choice you make. These aren't complicated rules to memorize—they're simple concepts that will become second nature once you understand the "why" behind them.

PRINCIPLE 1: NUTRIENT DENSE, NOT CALORIE DENSE

What Your Body Really Wants

Imagine your body as a high-performance car. You wouldn't put watered-down gasoline in a Ferrari, right? Yet that's essentially what we do when we eat calorie-dense but nutrient-poor foods. Your body needs premium fuel—foods packed with vitamins, minerals, antioxidants, and other compounds that support optimal function.

Nutrient Density Explained: Think of nutrient density as "nutrition per bite." It's the amount of beneficial nutrients you get relative to the calories consumed. A handful of spinach might have only 7 calories, but it's packed with folate, iron, vitamin K, and dozens of protective compounds. A handful of potato chips might have 150 calories but provides virtually no beneficial nutrients.

The Calorie Myth That's Making You Sick

Hernandez's Story: Hernandez meticulously counted calories and stayed within her daily limit, but she felt terrible. Her "diet" included diet sodas, low-fat processed snacks, and calorie-controlled frozen meals. Despite eating the "right" number of calories, she had constant cravings, energy crashes, and inflammatory symptoms. When she shifted to nutrient-dense whole foods—without counting a single calorie—her cravings disappeared, her energy stabilized, and she naturally reached her ideal weight.

❖ Why Calorie Counting Fails:
- Different foods trigger different hormonal responses

- Processed foods can cause inflammation regardless of calories
- Nutrient-poor foods leave you chronically hungry
- Your body's metabolism adjusts based on food quality, not just quantity

The Nutrient Density Hierarchy

- ❖ Tier 1: Super Nutrient Dense (Eat Abundantly)
- Leafy greens (spinach, kale, arugula)
- Colorful vegetables (bell peppers, broccoli, Brussels sprouts)
- Wild-caught fatty fish (salmon, sardines, mackerel)
- Organ meats (if you eat them)
- Berries and colorful fruits
- Nuts and seeds
- Herbs and spices

- ❖ Tier 2: Moderately Nutrient Dense (Eat Regularly)
- Whole grains (quinoa, brown rice, oats)
- Legumes (beans, lentils, chickpeas)
- Eggs from pasture-raised chickens
- Grass-fed meat and poultry
- Full-fat dairy from grass-fed animals
- Avocados and olives

- ❖ Tier 3: Lower Nutrient Density (Eat Occasionally)
- Refined grains (white rice, pasta)
- Natural sweeteners (honey, maple syrup)
- Conventional meat and dairy
- Processed foods with minimal ingredients

- ❖ Tier 4: Nutrient Poor/Inflammatory (Avoid or Minimize)
- Ultra-processed foods with long ingredient lists
- Foods with artificial additives
- Refined sugars and high-fructose corn syrup
- Trans fats and damaged oils
- Foods with inflammatory preservatives

Making Nutrient Density Practical

- ❖ The Plate Method:
- Fill half your plate with colorful vegetables
- One quarter with high-quality protein
- One quarter with nutrient-dense carbohydrates
- Add healthy fats throughout

The Crowding Out Strategy: Instead of focusing on what to eliminate, focus on adding more nutrient-dense foods. When you fill up on nourishing foods, you naturally have less room for inflammatory ones.

Example: Instead of saying "I can't eat chips," try "I'm going to have an apple with almond butter first." Often, after eating something truly nourishing, the craving for processed food diminishes or disappears entirely.

PRINCIPLE 2: BALANCING YOUR OMEGA OILS

The Fat That Changed Everything

In the 1950s, something unprecedented happened in human history: we began consuming massive amounts of omega-6 fatty acids while dramatically reducing omega-3 fatty acids. This shift has created one of the most significant inflammatory imbalances in our food supply.

The Omega Story: Your body needs both omega-3 and omega-6 fatty acids—they're essential, meaning your body can't make them. Think of them as two different types of chemical messengers:
- Omega-3s: Generally anti-inflammatory, calming, healing
- Omega-6s: Generally pro-inflammatory, but necessary for certain functions

The problem isn't that omega-6s are bad—it's that we're getting too many omega-6s and too few omega-3s.

The Great Omega Imbalance

- Historical Balance: Our ancestors consumed omega-6 to omega-3 in roughly a 1:1 to 4:1 ratio.

- Modern Imbalance: The average American now consumes omega-6 to omega-3 in a 20:1 to 50:1 ratio.

Why This Matters: These fatty acids compete for the same enzymes in your body. When omega-6s dominate, they crowd out omega-3s and promote inflammatory pathways.

Think of it like this Imagine your body's inflammatory response as a volume control. Omega-6s turn up the volume, while omega-3s turn it down. When the ratio is balanced, you have appropriate inflammatory responses. When it's imbalanced, the volume gets stuck on high.

The Omega-6 Overload

❖ Where Excess Omega-6s Hide:
- Vegetable oils (soybean, corn, sunflower, safflower oil)
- Processed foods made with these oils
- Conventionally raised meat and poultry (fed corn and soy)
- Fried foods and restaurant foods
- Packaged snacks and baked goods
- Salad dressings and mayonnaise

Lucas's Revelation: Lucas couldn't understand why his joint pain persisted despite eating "healthy" foods like grilled chicken and salads. The problem was subtle—he was cooking with vegetable oil and using store-bought dressings high in omega-6 oils. When he switched to olive oil and made his own dressings, his pain significantly decreased within weeks.

Omega-3 Powerhouses

❖ Marine Sources (Best Absorbed):
- Wild-caught salmon, sardines, mackerel, anchovies
- High-quality fish oil supplements
- Algae-based omega-3s (for vegetarians)

❖ Plant Sources:
- Flaxseeds and chia seeds
- Walnuts
- Hemp seeds
- Leafy greens (in smaller amounts)

Note: Plant-based omega-3s (ALA) need to be converted to the active forms (EPA and DHA) your body uses. This conversion is often inefficient, so marine sources are generally more effective.

Practical Omega Balancing

❖ Step 1: Reduce Omega-6 Intake
- Cook with olive oil, coconut oil, or avocado oil instead of vegetable oils
- Read labels and avoid products with soybean, corn, or sunflower oil
- Choose grass-fed meat when possible
- Limit fried and processed foods

❖ Step 2: Increase Omega-3 Intake
- Eat fatty fish 2-3 times per week
- Add ground flaxseed or chia seeds to smoothies
- Snack on walnuts instead of processed snacks
- Consider a high-quality fish oil supplement

❖ Step 3: Monitor Your Progress
- Pay attention to joint pain, skin health, and mood
- Consider omega-3 index testing if available
- Notice improvements in recovery from exercise

PRINCIPLE 3: ANTIOXIDANT SYNERGY AND PHYTONUTRIENT DIVERSITY

Free radicals are like sparks that can start fires in your body—they're unstable molecules that damage cells and promote inflammation. Antioxidants are like your body's internal fire department, neutralizing these harmful molecules before they can cause damage.

The Antioxidant Symphony: Here's something amazing: antioxidants work better together than individually. It's like a symphony orchestra—each instrument (antioxidant) is good on its own, but when they play together, the result is far more powerful than the sum of their parts.

The Color Code of Health

Nature has provided us with a simple way to ensure antioxidant diversity: eat a rainbow of colors. Each color represents different families of protective compounds:

❖ Red Foods:
- Tomatoes (lycopene)
- Berries (anthocyanins)
- Red peppers (capsanthin)
- Watermelon (lycopene)
Benefits: Heart health, cancer protection, eye health

❖ Orange/Yellow Foods:
- Carrots (beta-carotene)
- Sweet potatoes (beta-carotene)
- Turmeric (curcumin)
- Citrus fruits (vitamin C, flavonoids)
Benefits: Immune support, skin health, anti-inflammatory

❖ Green Foods:
- Leafy greens (chlorophyll, folate)
- Broccoli (sulforaphane)
- Green tea (catechins)
- Avocados (glutathione)
Benefits: Detoxification, cellular repair, brain health

❖ Blue/Purple Foods:
- Blueberries (anthocyanins)
- Eggplant (nasunin)
- Purple cabbage (anthocyanins)
- Grapes (resveratrol)
Benefits: Brain health, anti-aging, cardiovascular protection

❖ White/Tan Foods:
- Garlic (allicin)
- Onions (quercetin)
- Mushrooms (ergothioneine)
- Cauliflower (indoles)
Benefits: Immune support, detoxification, anti-microbial

The Phytonutrient Pharmacy

Plants produce thousands of protective compounds called phytonutrients. These aren't just antioxidants—they're sophisticated molecules that can:
- Modulate gene expression
- Support detoxification pathways
- Enhance immune function
- Protect against chronic diseases
- Reduce inflammation at the cellular level

The Diversity Principle: The more variety of plant foods you eat, the more diverse your phytonutrient intake. This is why eating 50 different fruits and vegetables per week is more beneficial than eating the same 5 over and over.

Maximizing Antioxidant Absorption

❖ Timing Matters:
- Eat antioxidant-rich foods with healthy fats (helps absorption of fat-soluble vitamins)
- Combine vitamin C foods with iron-rich foods (enhances iron absorption)
- Eat berries with yogurt or nuts (fats help antioxidant absorption)

❖ Preparation Matters:
- Lightly cooking tomatoes increases lycopene availability

- Crushing garlic and letting it sit activates beneficial compounds
- Eating berries fresh preserves heat-sensitive nutrients
- Combining turmeric with black pepper increases absorption

The Supplement vs. Food Debate

While supplements can be helpful, food sources of antioxidants are generally superior because:
- They provide synergistic compounds that work together
- They're better absorbed and utilized by your body
- They provide fiber and other beneficial nutrients
- They're less likely to cause imbalances

The 80/20 Rule: Aim to get 80% of your antioxidants from food sources, with supplements filling specific gaps based on your individual needs.

PRINCIPLE 4: GLYCEMIC LOAD MANAGEMENT

You've probably heard about avoiding sugar, but the reality is more nuanced. It's not just about the amount of sugar in food—it's about how quickly that food raises your blood sugar levels and how long those levels stay elevated.

Glycemic Load Explained: Think of glycemic load as the "blood sugar impact" of a food. It considers both the type of carbohydrate and the amount you're eating. A food can have a high glycemic index but a low glycemic load if you eat a small portion.

Why Blood Sugar Matters for Inflammation

The Blood Sugar Roller Coaster: When you eat high-glycemic foods, your blood sugar spikes rapidly. Your body responds by releasing insulin to bring it back down. But this creates a cascade of inflammatory responses:

1. Insulin Spikes: High insulin levels promote inflammation and fat storage
2. Glycation: Excess sugar binds to proteins, creating inflammatory compounds called AGEs (Advanced Glycation End-products)
3. Oxidative Stress: Blood sugar spikes generate free radicals that damage cells
4. Hormonal Disruption: Unstable blood sugar affects stress hormones and appetite regulation

Donald's Discovery: Donald couldn't understand why he felt anxious and irritable every afternoon around 3 PM. When he tracked his blood sugar patterns, he discovered that his breakfast of cereal and orange juice was causing a blood sugar crash exactly at that time. Switching to eggs and vegetables for breakfast eliminated his afternoon mood swings.

The Glycemic Load Hierarchy

❖ Low Glycemic Load (Eat Freely):
- Non-starchy vegetables
- Leafy greens
- Berries
- Nuts and seeds
- Protein foods
- Healthy fats

❖ Moderate Glycemic Load (Eat Mindfully):
- Whole grains
- Legumes
- Sweet potatoes
- Most fruits
- Dairy products

❖ High Glycemic Load (Eat Sparingly):
- White bread and refined grains
- Sugary drinks and desserts
- Processed breakfast cereals
- White potatoes (especially processed)
- Candy and sweets

Blood Sugar Balancing Strategies

❖ The Protein-Fat-Fiber Formula:
Every meal should include:
- Protein: Slows digestion and stabilizes blood sugar
- Healthy Fats: Further slow absorption and increase satiety
- Fiber: Moderates blood sugar response and feeds beneficial gut bacteria

❖ Meal Timing Strategies:
- Eat larger meals earlier in the day when insulin sensitivity is higher
- Avoid eating large amounts of carbohydrates late at night
- Consider intermittent fasting if appropriate for your lifestyle
- Don't skip meals (causes blood sugar instability)

❖ Food Combining Wisdom:
- Add vinegar to carbohydrate-rich meals (helps lower glycemic response)
- Eat protein before carbohydrates when possible
- Include cinnamon in sweet dishes (helps with blood sugar control)
- Choose whole fruits over fruit juices

Example: Instead of eating a banana alone (moderate glycemic load), eat it with almond butter (adds protein and fat) to significantly reduce the blood sugar impact.

PRINCIPLE 5: CIRCADIAN RHYTHM AND FOOD TIMING

Your body doesn't just process food—it processes it differently depending on the time of day. You have an internal clock (circadian rhythm) that influences everything from hormone production to digestive enzyme release.

❖ The Circadian Food Connection:
- Your insulin sensitivity is highest in the morning and lowest at night
- Digestive enzymes follow daily rhythms
- Melatonin production (your sleep hormone) is suppressed by late eating
- Your metabolism is most active during daylight hours

Timing Your Nutrition

- ❖ Morning (6 AM - 10 AM): Prime Time for Fuel
- Your body is most insulin-sensitive
- Cortisol levels are naturally higher (good for processing carbohydrates)
- Ideal time for larger meals with moderate carbohydrates
- Protein is especially important to stabilize blood sugar for the day

Optimal Morning Approach: Eat a substantial breakfast with protein, healthy fats, and some complex carbohydrates within 2 hours of waking.

- ❖ Midday (10 AM - 4 PM): Sustained Energy
- Continued good insulin sensitivity
- High digestive capacity
- Ideal time for your largest meal of the day
- Can handle moderate amounts of all macronutrients

Optimal Midday Approach: Make lunch your largest meal when possible, focusing on nutrient-dense whole foods.

- ❖ Evening (4 PM - 8 PM): Winding Down
- Insulin sensitivity begins to decline
- Digestive capacity decreases
- Melatonin production preparation begins
- Lighter meals are better processed

Optimal Evening Approach: Eat dinner at least 3 hours before bedtime, emphasizing protein and vegetables over heavy carbohydrates.

- ❖ Night (8 PM - 6 AM): Rest and Repair
- Lowest insulin sensitivity
- Digestive system needs rest
- Late eating disrupts sleep quality
- Fasting period allows cellular repair

Optimal Night Approach: Avoid eating 3 hours before bedtime. If you must eat, choose small amounts of easily digestible foods.

The Mediterranean Timing Wisdom

Traditional Mediterranean cultures have long practiced optimal meal timing:
- Breakfast: Moderate size, includes protein
- Lunch: Largest meal of the day, eaten leisurely
- Dinner: Lighter meal, eaten earlier in the evening
- Evening: Light socializing without heavy eating

This pattern aligns perfectly with our circadian biology and may explain part of the Mediterranean diet's health benefits.

Intermittent Fasting and Anti-Inflammatory Benefits

The Natural Fast: Humans naturally fast every night during sleep. Extending this fast can provide additional anti-inflammatory benefits:
- Allows digestive system to rest and repair
- Promotes cellular cleanup (autophagy)
- Improves insulin sensitivity
- Reduces overall inflammatory markers

❖ Simple Approaches:
- 12-hour window: Eat all meals within 12 hours (e.g., 7 AM to 7 PM)
- 16:8 method: Eat within 8 hours, fast for 16 hours
- Early time-restricted eating: Finish eating by 6 PM, break fast at 10 AM

Important Note: Intermittent fasting isn't appropriate for everyone. Pregnant women, people with eating disorders, and those with certain medical conditions should consult healthcare providers first.

PUTTING IT ALL TOGETHER: YOUR ANTI-INFLAMMATORY EATING FOUNDATION

These five principles don't work in isolation—they work together to create a powerful anti-inflammatory effect:

1. Nutrient density ensures your body gets what it needs to function optimally
2. Balanced omegas provide the right building blocks for healthy inflammatory responses
3. Antioxidant diversity protects your cells from damage and supports healing
4. Glycemic control prevents inflammatory blood sugar spikes
5. Proper timing aligns your eating with your body's natural rhythms

Your 30-Day Foundation Challenge

❖ Week 1: Nutrient Density Focus
- Add one extra serving of vegetables to each meal
- Replace one processed snack with a whole food option
- Try one new colorful fruit or vegetable

❖ Week 2: Omega Balance
- Switch cooking oils to olive or avocado oil
- Add fatty fish twice this week
- Include nuts or seeds as snacks

❖ Week 3: Antioxidant Rainbow
- Eat at least 5 different colored foods daily
- Add herbs and spices to every meal
- Try one new antioxidant-rich food

❖ Week 4: Timing and Glycemic Control
- Eat your largest meal at lunch
- Stop eating 3 hours before bedtime
- Combine proteins and fats with any carbohydrates

Measuring Your Success

- ❖ Track These Improvements:
- Energy levels throughout the day
- Sleep quality and ease of falling asleep
- Mood stability and mental clarity
- Digestive comfort and regularity
- Joint pain or stiffness levels
- Skin clarity and appearance
- Cravings for processed foods
- Overall sense of well-being

Remember: Progress, Not Perfection

- The 80/20 Principle: Aim to follow these principles 80% of the time. The 20% flexibility allows for social situations, travel, and life's unexpected moments without derailing your progress.

- Start Where You Are: You don't need to implement all five principles perfectly from day one. Choose the one that resonates most with you and build from there.

- Listen to Your Body: These are guidelines, not rigid rules. Pay attention to how different foods and timing patterns affect you personally.

When you understand the principles behind healthy eating, you don't need to follow diet rules—you become the expert on what your body needs.

Chapter 6 Key Takeaways

The Five Core Principles**:
1. Nutrient Density: Choose foods that provide maximum nutrition per calorie
2. Omega Balance: Optimize your omega-3 to omega-6 ratio for reduced inflammation
3. Antioxidant Synergy: Eat a rainbow of colors to maximize protective compounds
4. Glycemic Control: Manage blood sugar responses to prevent inflammatory spikes
5. Circadian Timing: Align your eating patterns with your body's natural rhythms

What You Can Do Today:
- Use the Anti-Inflammatory Food Pyramid to plan your next meal
- Add one new colorful vegetable to your shopping list
- Replace one cooking oil with olive oil or avocado oil
- Plan to eat your largest meal earlier in the day
- Start your 30-day foundation challenge with Week 1 goals

PART III

BEYOND THE PLATE ~ LIFESTYLE INTEGRATION

Chapter 7

Stress Management and Inflammation

The same mind that created your stress has the power to dissolve it. Your breath is the key that unlocks this power.

Here's something that might surprise you: your thoughts and emotions have a direct, measurable impact on the inflammatory chemicals circulating in your bloodstream. Within minutes of experiencing stress, anxiety, or anger, your body begins producing inflammatory compounds that can affect every organ system.

But here's the empowering truth: just as negative emotions can trigger inflammation, positive mental states and stress-reduction techniques can powerfully reduce it. In this chapter, you'll learn how to harness your mind's incredible ability to heal your body from the inside out.

You don't need years of meditation training or expensive retreats. You need practical, science-backed techniques that fit into your real life and start working immediately. Let's begin by understanding exactly how your stress response affects your health, then dive into the most effective tools for taking control.

THE CORTISOL-INFLAMMATION CONNECTION: YOUR BODY'S INTERNAL ALARM SYSTEM

Imagine your body has an internal security system with motion sensors, cameras, and alarms. This is your stress response system, and it's designed to protect you from danger. When it works properly, it's brilliant. When it gets stuck in "alarm mode," it becomes your biggest health challenge.

The Acute Stress Response (How It Should Work):
1. Threat Detection: Your brain perceives danger (real or imagined)
2. Alarm Activation: Your hypothalamus triggers the release of stress hormones
3. Body Mobilization: Cortisol and adrenaline flood your system
4. Enhanced Performance: You become stronger, faster, and more alert
5. Threat Resolution: You handle the situation
6. System Reset: Stress hormones return to normal levels
7. Recovery: Your body repairs and restores itself

This system saved your ancestors from predators and still helps you in true emergencies. The problem? Your modern life activates this system dozens of times per day for non-life-threatening situations.

When Your Alarm System Breaks

❖ Modern Stress Triggers:
- Work deadlines and pressure
- Financial concerns
- Relationship conflicts
- Traffic jams and commuting

- Social media and news consumption
- Health worries
- Parenting challenges
- Technology overwhelm
- Information overload
- Comparison and competition

Your brain can't distinguish between a charging lion and a demanding boss. Both trigger the same stress response, flooding your body with inflammatory chemicals.

The Inflammatory Cascade of Chronic Stress

When stress becomes chronic, here's what happens in your body:

❖ Cortisol Dysregulation:
- Normal Pattern: Cortisol should be high in the morning (to wake you up) and low at night (to help you sleep)
- Stressed Pattern: Cortisol remains elevated throughout the day or becomes completely depleted
- Inflammatory Impact: Chronically elevated cortisol directly increases inflammatory markers in your blood

❖ The Vicious Cycle:
1. Stress triggers cortisol release
2. Cortisol initially suppresses inflammation (which is why you might feel "wired but tired")
3. Chronic cortisol elevation eventually leads to cortisol resistance
4. Your body loses its ability to control inflammation naturally
5. Inflammation increases, making you more sensitive to stress
6. Increased stress sensitivity triggers more cortisol release
7. The cycle continues, getting worse over time

Real Example: Jennifer, a marketing director, lived in constant stress for two years. She developed mysterious joint pain, digestive issues, frequent colds, and insomnia. Multiple doctors found nothing wrong in her tests. When she finally addressed her chronic stress through the techniques in this chapter, all her symptoms gradually resolved. "I didn't realize my mind was literally making my body sick," she said.

The Physical Toll of Mental Stress

Chronic stress doesn't just make you feel anxious—it creates measurable physical changes:

❖ Immediate Effects (Within Minutes to Hours):
- Increased heart rate and blood pressure
- Elevated blood sugar levels
- Suppressed digestion
- Heightened inflammation markers
- Reduced immune function

❖ Short-term Effects (Days to Weeks):
- Disrupted sleep patterns
- Digestive problems
- Frequent infections
- Muscle tension and pain
- Mood swings and irritability

❖ Long-term Effects (Months to Years):
- Cardiovascular disease
- Autoimmune conditions
- Diabetes and metabolic syndrome
- Depression and anxiety disorders
- Accelerated aging
- Increased cancer risk

The Hopeful Truth: These effects are largely reversible. When you learn to manage stress effectively, your body begins healing almost immediately.

MINDFULNESS-BASED STRESS REDUCTION: YOUR MENTAL RESET BUTTON

Mindfulness isn't about emptying your mind or sitting in uncomfortable positions. It's simply about paying attention to the present moment without judgment. Think of it as giving your overactive mind a chance to rest and reset.

❖ The Science is Clear:
- Just 8 weeks of mindfulness practice can measurably reduce inflammatory markers
- Mindfulness meditation changes brain structure in areas related to stress and emotion regulation
- Regular practice lowers cortisol levels and improves immune function
- People who practice mindfulness have lower rates of heart disease, depression, and chronic pain

Practical Mindfulness for Busy Lives

❖ The 3-Minute Reset (Perfect for Beginners):
1. Minute 1 - Notice: Sit comfortably and simply notice what you're thinking and feeling without trying to change anything
2. Minute 2 - Breathe: Focus on your breath, noticing each inhale and exhale
3. Minute 3 - Expand: Expand your awareness to include your whole body and surrounding environment

Mindful Daily Activities: You don't need extra time—just bring mindfulness to activities you already do:

- Mindful Eating: Pay attention to flavors, textures, and how food makes you feel
- Mindful Walking: Notice your steps, surroundings, and breath while walking
- Mindful Listening: Give full attention to conversations without planning your response
- Mindful Cleaning: Focus on the sensations and movements of household tasks
- Mindful Commuting: Use travel time for breathing exercises or gentle awareness

Advanced Mindfulness Techniques

❖ Body Scan Meditation (10-20 minutes):
This practice helps you reconnect with your body and release stored tension:
1. Lie down comfortably
2. Starting with your toes, slowly move your attention through each part of your body
3. Notice any sensations without trying to change them
4. Breathe into areas of tension or discomfort
5. End by noticing your body as a whole

Loving-Kindness Meditation (Especially powerful for reducing inflammation):

Research shows that cultivating positive emotions toward yourself and others significantly reduces inflammatory markers:
1. Begin by sending kind wishes to yourself: "May I be happy, may I be healthy, may I be at peace"
2. Extend these wishes to loved ones
3. Include neutral people in your life
4. Even include difficult people (this is advanced but incredibly healing)
5. Finish by sending kindness to all living beings

BREATHING EXERCISES: YOUR BUILT-IN ANTI-INFLAMMATORY MEDICINE

The Breath-Inflammation Connection

Your breath is the most powerful tool you have for instantly shifting from stress mode to healing mode. Unlike your heart rate or blood pressure, you can consciously control your breathing, and this control directly impacts your nervous system and inflammation levels.

- ❖ How Breathing Affects Inflammation:
- Deep, slow breathing activates your parasympathetic nervous system (rest and digest mode)
- This reduces cortisol production and inflammatory chemical release
- Improved oxygenation helps your body's natural detoxification processes
- Rhythmic breathing helps synchronize your heart rate variability, a marker of resilience

The Most Effective Anti-Inflammatory Breathing Techniques

- ❖ The 4-7-8 Breath (Instantly calming):

Perfect for acute stress or before sleep:
1. Exhale completely through your mouth
2. Inhale through your nose for 4 counts
3. Hold your breath for 7 counts
4. Exhale through your mouth for 8 counts
5. Repeat 3-4 times

Why it works: The extended exhale activates your parasympathetic nervous system, immediately reducing stress hormone production.

- ❖ Box Breathing (For focus and calm):

Used by Navy SEALs and emergency responders:
1. Inhale for 4 counts
2. Hold for 4 counts
3. Exhale for 4 counts
4. Hold empty for 4 counts
5. Repeat for 5-10 cycles

When to use: Before stressful meetings, during traffic, or anytime you need to center yourself.

- ❖ Coherent Breathing (For long-term resilience):

This technique optimizes heart rate variability:
1. Breathe in for 5 counts
2. Breathe out for 5 counts
3. Continue for 10-20 minutes
4. Practice daily for best results

❖ The Anti-Inflammatory Breath (My personal favorite):
This technique specifically targets inflammation reduction:
1. Inhale slowly through your nose, imagining healing energy entering your body
2. Hold briefly while visualizing this energy reaching areas of pain or inflammation
3. Exhale slowly through your mouth, imagining stress and inflammation leaving your body
4. Repeat 10-15 times

Breathing Throughout Your Day

❖ Micro-Breathing Breaks:
- Take 3 deep breaths before checking email
- Use red lights as reminders to breathe deeply
- Breathe consciously while waiting in lines
- Take 5 deep breaths before eating meals
- End each hour with 1 minute of focused breathing

The 5-5-5 Rule: Every 5 hours, take 5 minutes for 5 deep breaths. This simple practice can significantly reduce your daily inflammatory load.

NATURE THERAPY: THE HEALING POWER OF THE OUTDOORS

Forest Bathing: Medicine from Trees

In Japan, "forest bathing" (shinrin-yoku) is actually prescribed by doctors. It's not about hiking or exercising—it's about mindfully immersing yourself in nature using all your senses.

❖ The Science Behind Nature's Anti-Inflammatory Effects:
- Trees release airborne chemicals called phytoncides that boost immune function
- Natural environments reduce cortisol levels more effectively than indoor relaxation
- Exposure to sunlight helps regulate circadian rhythms and vitamin D production
- Natural sounds mask urban noise stress
- Green spaces encourage physical activity and social connection

❖ Research Findings:
- Just 15 minutes in nature can significantly reduce inflammatory markers
- Hospital patients with views of trees heal faster than those with urban views
- Children who spend time in nature have lower rates of attention disorders and anxiety
- Adults who live near green spaces have lower rates of heart disease and depression

Practical Nature Therapy for Urban Dwellers

❖ You Don't Need a Forest:
- City parks and tree-lined streets provide benefits
- Even looking at nature photographs can reduce stress hormones
- Indoor plants improve air quality and reduce stress
- Water features (fountains, aquariums) create calming environments

❖ Micro-Nature Experiences:
- The 5-Minute Garden: Step outside and mindfully observe plants, sky, or weather
- Window Gazing: Look out windows at natural elements during work breaks

- Barefoot Grounding: Stand barefoot on grass or earth for a few minutes
- Weather Watching: Consciously notice and appreciate weather changes
- Star Gazing: Look up at the sky, even in urban areas

David's Routine: David, a software developer who worked 60-hour weeks, started taking 10-minute walks in a nearby park every lunch break. This simple practice reduced his chronic headaches and improved his afternoon productivity. "I didn't realize how much I needed that nature break," he said.

Advanced Nature Therapy Techniques

❖ Forest Bathing Practice (2-4 hours when possible):
1. Enter a natural area with intention to be present
2. Turn off devices and distractions
3. Walk very slowly, stopping frequently
4. Engage all senses: touch bark, smell flowers, listen to birds
5. Sit quietly for extended periods
6. Breathe deeply and consciously
7. Leave feeling refreshed and restored

❖ Seasonal Nature Connection:
- Spring: Notice new growth and renewal
- Summer: Appreciate abundance and vitality
- Fall: Observe change and letting go
- Winter: Find beauty in stillness and rest

❖ Nature Journaling: Writing about nature experiences amplifies their anti-inflammatory benefits:
- Describe what you see, hear, smell, and feel
- Note how nature experiences affect your mood and energy
- Track patterns between nature time and physical symptoms
- Express gratitude for natural beauty

SOCIAL CONNECTION: YOUR IMMUNE SYSTEM'S BEST FRIEND

Humans are wired for connection. Loneliness and social isolation trigger inflammatory responses similar to physical injury. Your body interprets social rejection as a threat to survival and responds accordingly.

❖ The Loneliness-Inflammation Connection:
- Social isolation increases inflammatory markers by up to 30%
- Loneliness is as harmful to health as smoking 15 cigarettes per day
- People with strong social connections have 50% better survival rates from serious illness
- Social support directly reduces cortisol production and inflammatory responses

Quality vs. Quantity: It's not about having hundreds of friends—it's about having meaningful connections where you feel seen, heard, and valued.

Building Anti-Inflammatory Relationships

❖ Characteristics of Healing Relationships:
- Safety: You can be yourself without fear of judgment
- Support: Others offer help during difficult times
- Reciprocity: Relationships involve mutual giving and receiving

- Authenticity: You can share both struggles and joys
- Growth: Relationships encourage personal development
- Fun: You enjoy spending time together

❖ Toxic Relationships and Inflammation:
Some relationships actually increase inflammation:
- Constant criticism or judgment
- Emotional manipulation or control
- Lack of reciprocity (all giving or all taking)
- Drama and conflict without resolution
- Feeling drained rather than energized after interactions

Practical Strategies for Social Anti-Inflammatory Health

❖ Building New Connections:
- Join groups based on interests (hiking, cooking, and book clubs)
- Volunteer for causes you care about
- Take classes or workshops
- Attend community events
- Use apps designed for friend-making (like Meetup or Bumble BFF)
- Say yes to social invitations, even when you don't feel like it

❖ Deepening Existing Relationships:
- Schedule regular one-on-one time with people you care about
- Practice active listening without trying to fix or advice
- Share vulnerable thoughts and feelings appropriately
- Express gratitude and appreciation regularly
- Create rituals and traditions together
- Support others during their difficult times

❖ The Anti-Inflammatory Conversation:
How you talk with others affects your inflammatory levels:
- Gossiping and complaining increase stress hormones
- Expressing gratitude and appreciation reduce inflammatory markers
- Sharing positive experiences boost immune function
- Offering and receiving support lower cortisol levels
- Laughing together is one of the most powerful anti-inflammatory activities

Digital Connection vs. Real Connection

❖ The Social Media Paradox: While social media can help maintain connections, it often increases rather than decreases loneliness and inflammation:
- Comparison and FOMO (fear of missing out) trigger stress responses
- Passive scrolling doesn't provide the benefits of real interaction
- Online conflict and negativity increase inflammatory markers
- Screen time often replaces face-to-face connection

❖ Healthy Digital Boundaries:
- Use technology to facilitate real-world connections
- Limit passive social media consumption
- Curate feeds to include more positive, inspiring content

- Have device-free times for in-person interactions
- Use video calls when face-to-face isn't possible

PRACTICAL TOOL: THE 21-DAY STRESS REDUCTION PROTOCOL

This comprehensive program combines all the techniques in this chapter into a progressive, manageable plan. Each week builds on the previous one, creating lasting habits that will transform your stress response and reduce inflammation.

Week 1: Foundation Building

- ❖ Daily Practices:
- Morning: 5 minutes of mindful breathing upon waking
- Midday: 3-minute mindfulness reset during lunch
- Evening: 10 minutes of body scan meditation before bed

- ❖ Weekly Challenges:
- Day 1-2: Identify your top 3 stress triggers
- Day 3-4: Practice the 4-7-8 breath during each trigger
- Day 5-6: Spend 15 minutes in nature daily
- Day 7: Reflect on the week and adjust practices as needed

Tracking: Rate your stress level (1-10) and note physical symptoms daily

Week 2: Expansion and Integration

- ❖ Daily Practices:
- Continue Week 1 practices
- Add one mindful daily activity (eating, walking, or cleaning)
- Include 5 minutes of loving-kindness meditation
- Take three 2-minute breathing breaks throughout the day

- ❖ Weekly Challenges:
- Day 8-9: Try forest bathing or extended nature time
- Day 10-11: Reach out to one person for meaningful connection
- Day 12-13: Practice boundary-setting with one stressful situation
- Day 14: Have a completely screen-free evening

Tracking: Continue stress rating and add energy levels and mood

Week 3: Mastery and Sustainability

- ❖ Daily Practices:
- Choose your 3 favorite practices from Weeks 1-2
- Add coherent breathing practice (10-20 minutes)
- Implement the 5-5-5 breathing rule
- Practice gratitude journaling (3 things daily)

- ❖ Weekly Challenges:
- Day 15-16: Organize a social activity with friends or family

- Day 17-18: Create a nature space in your home or office
- Day 19-20: Practice advanced mindfulness during a typically stressful situation
- Day 21: Design your sustainable long-term stress management plan

Tracking: Note which practices are most effective for you

Daily Tracking Sheet (Print or copy this format)

*Date: _____
*Overall Stress Level (1-10): ___
*Energy Level (1-10): ___
*Mood (1-10): ___
*Sleep Quality (1-10): ___

- ❖ Practices Completed Today:
- ☐ Morning breathing/mindfulness
- ☐ Midday reset
- ☐ Evening relaxation
- ☐ Nature time
- ☐ Social connection
- ☐ Physical symptoms: _____

*What worked best today: _____
*What was challenging: _____
*Tomorrow's intention: _____

Customization Options

- ❖ For Busy Schedules:
- Focus on micro-practices (1-3 minutes)
- Use commute time for breathing exercises
- Combine practices (mindful walking, breathing in nature)
- Prioritize consistency over duration

- ❖ For High-Stress Periods:
- Increase breathing exercises frequency
- Add emergency stress-relief techniques
- Seek additional social support
- Consider professional help if needed

- ❖ For Social Introverts:
- Start with one-on-one connections
- Use nature time as social space
- Focus more on deepening existing relationships
- Remember that even small social interactions help

ADVANCED STRESS MANAGEMENT STRATEGIES

Everyone responds differently to stress-reduction techniques. Create a personalized toolkit with your most effective strategies:

❖ Immediate Relief (for acute stress):
- Emergency breathing technique
- Progressive muscle relaxation
- Cold water on face and wrists
- Essential oils or calming scents
- Soothing music or sounds

❖ Daily Maintenance (for ongoing resilience):
- Morning mindfulness routine
- Regular exercise or movement
- Consistent sleep schedule
- Nutritious anti-inflammatory meals
- Time in nature

❖ Weekly Restoration (for deeper healing):
- Extended nature time
- Social activities with loved ones
- Creative or recreational activities
- Massage or other bodywork
- Spiritual or contemplative practices

Stress Inoculation Training

Just as vaccines help your immune system handle pathogens, you can train your stress response system to handle challenges more effectively:

❖ Gradual Exposure:
- Purposefully engage in mildly challenging situations
- Practice stress-reduction techniques during low-stress times
- Build confidence through small successes
- Gradually increase challenges as resilience improves

❖ Mental Rehearsal:
- Visualize handling stressful situations calmly
- Practice your coping strategies mentally
- Imagine successful outcomes
- Prepare responses to common stressors

When to Seek Professional Help

While self-care strategies are powerful, sometimes additional support is needed:

❖ Consider Professional Help If:
- Stress significantly impacts daily functioning
- Physical symptoms persist despite lifestyle changes
- You experience anxiety or depression
- Relationships are suffering due to stress
- You use alcohol, drugs, or other substances to cope
- Sleep problems persist despite good sleep hygiene

❖ Types of Professional Support:
- Cognitive-behavioral therapy (CBT)
- Mindfulness-based stress reduction (MBSR) programs
- Biofeedback training
- Massage therapy or acupuncture
- Support groups
- Medical evaluation for underlying conditions

CREATING YOUR ANTI-INFLAMMATORY LIFESTYLE

Integration with Other Healthy Habits

Stress management works best when integrated with other anti-inflammatory practices:

❖ Synergistic Effects:
- Exercise reduces stress hormones and improves mood
- Anti-inflammatory foods support stable energy and mood
- Good sleep improves stress resilience
- Social connections provide practical and emotional support
- Nature time combines movement, mindfulness, and social opportunities

Making It Sustainable

*Start Small: Begin with just one or two techniques that appeal to you most
*Be Consistent: Daily practice, even for short periods, is more effective than occasional longer sessions
*Stay Flexible: Adapt practices to changing circumstances and needs
*Track Progress: Notice improvements in mood, energy, sleep, and physical symptoms
*Celebrate Success: Acknowledge positive changes, no matter how small

Remember: The goal isn't to eliminate all stress from your life—that's impossible and wouldn't be healthy. The goal is to develop a healthy relationship with stress where you can respond rather than react, recover quickly, and maintain your physical and emotional well-being even during challenging times.

Your Stress-Inflammation Success Metrics

Track these markers to measure your progress:

❖ Subjective Measures:
- Daily stress levels (1-10 scale)
- Energy and mood ratings
- Sleep quality assessments
- Physical symptom tracking
- Overall sense of well-being

❖ Objective Measures (if available):
- Resting heart rate and blood pressure
- Heart rate variability (using apps or devices)
- Inflammatory markers (CRP, IL-6) through blood tests
- Cortisol patterns (saliva tests)
- Sleep quality metrics (from sleep tracking devices)

Your Stress-Free Future

Imagine waking up tomorrow feeling calm and centered, regardless of what your day might bring. Picture yourself handling challenges with grace, sleeping peacefully at night, and feeling genuinely connected to the people around you. This isn't a fantasy—it's the natural state of a nervous system that's been trained to respond rather than react.

The techniques in this chapter aren't just tools for managing stress—they're pathways to a fundamentally different way of being in the world. When you commit to these practices, you're not just reducing inflammation—you're reclaiming your power to shape your own experience of life.

Every breath you take consciously, every moment you spend in mindful awareness, every connection you nurture with another person is an investment in your long-term health and happiness. The inflammation-reducing effects are just the beginning. You're building resilience, wisdom, and a deep sense of inner peace that no external circumstance can shake.

Start today. Start small. Start where you are. Your calmer, healthier, more connected future self is waiting.

Peace is not the absence of conflict, but the ability to cope with it calmly and effectively

Chapter 9 Key Takeaways

- ❖ What You Learned:
- Chronic stress directly increases inflammatory markers through cortisol dysregulation
- Mindfulness, breathing exercises, nature therapy, and social connection are scientifically proven to reduce inflammation
- Your stress response can be retrained through consistent practice
- Small, daily practices are more effective than occasional intensive efforts
- Social connections are as important to health as diet and exercise

- ❖ What You Can Do Right Now:
- Try the 4-7-8 breathing technique the next time you feel stressed
- Schedule 10 minutes of nature time into your day
- Reach out to one person for meaningful connection
- Begin the 21-Day Stress Reduction Protocol
- Identify your top 3 stress triggers and choose one breathing technique to use with each

Chapter 8

Environmental Detoxification

Your home should be a place where your body heals, not where it struggles to survive. Every small change you make creates a ripple effect of wellness throughout your daily life.

Picture this: You wake up and immediately breathe in air freshener chemicals. You shower with products containing endocrine disruptors. You clean your teeth with fluoride and artificial colors. You drink water with chlorine and pharmaceutical residues. You eat breakfast off plates containing BPA. You clean your counters with antibacterial chemicals. And you haven't even left your house yet.

This isn't meant to scare you—it's meant to wake you up to the reality that your body is working incredibly hard just to process the chemical soup of modern living. But here's the empowering truth: you have more control over your environment than you realize, and small, strategic changes can dramatically reduce your inflammatory burden.

Understanding your Toxic Load

Think of your body as a bucket that collects toxins throughout the day. Everyone's bucket has a different capacity based on genetics, age, overall health, and detoxification ability. When your bucket is only half full, you might not notice any symptoms. But when it starts to overflow, that's when inflammation, fatigue, headaches, and other health issues appear.

- ❖ Your Daily Toxic Sources:
- Indoor Air: Often 2-5 times more polluted than outdoor air
- Water: Contains chlorine, fluoride, pharmaceutical residues, and heavy metals
- Personal Care Products: Average woman uses 168 chemicals daily before breakfast
- Household Cleaners: Release volatile organic compounds (VOCs) that linger for hours
- Food Packaging: BPA, phthalates, and other chemicals leach into food
- Furniture and Carpets: Off-gas formaldehyde and flame retardants for years

The Good News: Unlike genetics, you have direct control over most of these exposure sources. Reducing your daily toxic load is like poking holes in the bottom of your bucket—your body can handle reasonable exposure when it's not overwhelmed.

AIR QUALITY: YOUR MOST IMPORTANT ENVIRONMENT

You can survive weeks without food, days without water, but only minutes without air. Yet most people pay more attention to their food quality than their air quality, despite breathing over 20,000 times per day.

The Hidden Dangers in Your Air

- ❖ Indoor Air Pollutants:
- Volatile Organic Compounds (VOCs): From paints, furniture, cleaning products

- Formaldehyde: Released from pressed wood, carpets, and fabrics
- Flame Retardants: From furniture, electronics, and textiles
- Mold and Mycotoxins: From moisture damage and poor ventilation
- Particulate Matter: From cooking, candles, and outdoor pollution
- Chemical Fragrances: From air fresheners, candles, and cleaning products

Real Story: Jane couldn't figure out why she always felt tired and congested at home but felt better at work and outdoors. An air quality test revealed high levels of formaldehyde from her new furniture and VOCs from scented candles she burned daily. Within two weeks of removing these sources and improving ventilation, her energy returned and her chronic sinus issues resolved.

Immediate Air Quality Improvements

❖ The Fresh Air Foundation:
1. Open Windows Daily: Even 5-10 minutes of fresh air exchange can dramatically improve indoor air quality
2. Create Cross-Ventilation: Open windows on opposite sides of your home to create airflow
3. Use Exhaust Fans: Run bathroom and kitchen fans during and after use
4. Avoid Synthetic Fragrances: Eliminate air fresheners, scented candles, and plug-in air fresheners

Natural Air Purification: Plants aren't just decorative—they're living air purifiers. NASA research identified plants that effectively remove common indoor pollutants:

❖ Top Air-Purifying Plants:
- Snake Plant: Removes formaldehyde and benzene, produces oxygen at night
- Spider Plant: Eliminates formaldehyde and xylene
- Peace Lily: Removes ammonia, benzene, and formaldehyde
- Boston Fern: Naturally humidifies air and removes formaldehyde
- Rubber Plant: Removes formaldehyde and is very low-maintenance

Placement Strategy: One plant per 100 square feet of living space provides measurable air quality improvement.

❖ Mechanical Air Purification: If you're dealing with significant air quality issues, consider an air purifier with:
- HEPA Filter: Removes 99.97% of particles 0.3 microns or larger
- Activated Carbon: Absorbs chemicals, odors, and VOCs
- Appropriate Size: Should cycle room air 4-6 times per hour

❖ Budget-Friendly Air Quality Hacks:
- Beeswax Candles: Unlike paraffin candles, these actually purify air
- Salt Lamps: May help reduce positive ions and electromagnetic pollution
- Activated Charcoal Bags: Natural odor and moisture absorbers
- Essential Oil Diffusers: Use pure essential oils instead of synthetic fragrances

Specific Air Quality Strategies

❖ For Cooking Pollution:
- Always use exhaust fans when cooking
- Choose lower-heat cooking methods when possible
- Avoid non-stick cookware that releases toxins when heated
- Open windows during and after cooking

❖ For Bedroom Air Quality:

- Keep bedroom doors open during the day for air circulation
- Avoid synthetic bedding materials that off-gas chemicals
- Remove electronics from the bedroom (they emit heat and electromagnetic fields)
- Use natural fiber bedding and pajamas

❖ For Home Office Air Quality:
- Position your workspace near a window
- Add plants specifically for your workspace
- Avoid synthetic office furniture when possible
- Take regular fresh air breaks

WATER: THE FOUNDATION OF CELLULAR HEALTH

Water makes up 60% of your body and is involved in every cellular process. The quality of your water directly impacts the quality of your health, yet most people put more thought into their car's fuel than their body's primary fuel.

What's Really in Your Water

❖ Common Tap Water Contaminants:
- Chlorine: Added for disinfection but disrupts gut bacteria and can form carcinogenic byproducts
- Fluoride: Added to prevent tooth decay but accumulates in tissues and may disrupt thyroid function
- Heavy Metals: Lead, mercury, and arsenic from old pipes and environmental contamination
- Pharmaceutical Residues: Birth control hormones, antibiotics, and antidepressants
- Pesticides and Herbicides: Agricultural runoff containing endocrine disruptors
- Microplastics: Tiny plastic particles found in most water supplies

Tom's Discovery: Tom struggled with digestive issues for years. When he installed a quality water filter, his bloating and irregular bowel movements improved within weeks. "I didn't realize how much the chlorine in my water was affecting my gut bacteria," he said.

Water Filtration Solutions

Understanding Your Options:

❖ Carbon Filters (Good for most people):
- Remove chlorine, odors, and many chemicals
- Improve taste significantly
- Relatively inexpensive
- Don't remove minerals (which is good)
- Examples: Brita, PUR, under-sink carbon systems

❖ Reverse Osmosis (For heavily contaminated water):
- Removes almost everything, including heavy metals and fluoride
- More expensive but very thorough
- Removes beneficial minerals (consider remineralization)
- Slower filtration process
- Best for areas with known water quality problems

❖ Whole House Systems (For comprehensive protection):
- Filter all water entering your home

- Protect skin and lungs from chlorine during showers
- Higher upfront cost but protect entire family
- Reduce need for individual filters throughout house

❖ Simple Starting Points:
1. Get Your Water Tested: Many areas offer free testing, or you can purchase test kits online
2. Start with a Counter-Top Filter: Affordable way to immediately improve drinking water
3. Filter Shower Water: A simple shower filter can reduce chlorine exposure through your skin and lungs
4. Upgrade Gradually: Start with drinking water, then expand to whole house as budget allows

Hydration Optimization

Quality + Quantity + Timing = Optimal Hydration

❖ How Much Water Do You Really Need?
The "8 glasses a day" rule is overly simplistic. Your needs depend on:
- Body size and activity level
- Climate and season
- Overall health status
- Caffeine and alcohol consumption
- Medication use

A Better Formula: Drink half your body weight in ounces, plus 12-16 ounces for every hour of exercise or high heat exposure.

❖ Hydration Timing Strategies:
- Upon Waking: 16-20 ounces to rehydrate after hours without water
- Before Meals: 8-16 ounces 30 minutes before eating aids digestion
- During Exercise: 4-6 ounces every 15-20 minutes during activity
- Evening Taper: Reduce intake 2-3 hours before bed to avoid sleep disruption

❖ Signs You're Properly Hydrated:
- Urine is pale yellow (not clear, not dark)
- You rarely feel thirsty
- Energy levels are stable throughout the day
- Skin has good elasticity
- You're not getting frequent headaches

❖ Hydration Enhancers:
- Add Minerals: A pinch of high-quality sea salt or electrolyte powder
- Infuse Naturally: Cucumber, lemon, mint, or berries for flavor without chemicals
- Room Temperature: Easier for your body to absorb than ice-cold water
- Glass Containers: Avoid plastic bottles that can leach chemicals

PERSONAL CARE PRODUCTS: WHAT YOU PUT ON YOUR BODY GOES IN YOUR BODY

Your skin is your largest organ and absorbs much of what you put on it. The average woman uses 168 different chemicals in her daily beauty routine—before breakfast. Many of these chemicals are endocrine disruptors that interfere with hormone function and trigger inflammation.

The Dirty Dozen: Ingredients to Avoid

❖ Immediate Red Flags:
1. Parabens (methylparaben, propylparaben): Hormone disruptors linked to breast cancer
2. Phthalates (often hidden in "fragrance"): Reproductive toxins and hormone disruptors
3. Sodium Lauryl Sulfate (SLS): Skin irritant that can cause inflammation
4. Formaldehyde-Releasing Preservatives: Known carcinogens
5. Synthetic Fragrances: Can contain hundreds of unlisted chemicals
6. Triclosan: Antibacterial agent that disrupts microbiome and hormones
7. Aluminum (in antiperspirants): Potential neurotoxin and hormone disruptor
8. Petroleum-Based Ingredients: Can contain carcinogenic impurities
9. Synthetic Colors (FD&C, D&C numbers): Many are carcinogenic
10. Diethanolamine (DEA): Carcinogenic when combined with nitrates
11. Butylated Hydroxytoluene (BHT): Potential carcinogen and hormone disruptor
12. Oxybenzone (in sunscreens): Hormone disruptor absorbed through skin

Reading Labels Like a Pro

❖ Red Flag Words to Avoid:
- "Fragrance" or "Parfum" (can hide hundreds of chemicals)
- Long chemical names you can't pronounce
- Numbers after ingredient names (usually synthetic)
- "Antibacterial" (often contains triclosan)

❖ Green Flag Words to Look For:
- "Organic" (when certified)
- "Plant-based" or "Botanical"
- "Fragrance-free" (not "unscented")
- "Non-toxic" or "Natural"
- Recognizable plant names

Simple Swaps for Every Product

❖ Cleansers and Soaps:
- Instead of: Harsh antibacterial soaps with triclosan
- Choose: Castile soap, gentle plant-based cleansers, or simple bar soaps
- DIY Option: Mix castile soap with honey and essential oils

❖ Shampoo and Conditioner:
- Instead of: Sulfate-laden shampoos with synthetic fragrances
- Choose: Sulfate-free, naturally scented options
- Natural Alternative: Apple cider vinegar rinse, coconut oil treatments

❖ Deodorant:
- Instead of: Aluminum-based antiperspirants
- Choose: Natural deodorants with baking soda, arrowroot, or magnesium
- Transition Tip: It takes 2-4 weeks for your body to adjust to natural deodorant

❖ Moisturizers and Lotions:
- Instead of: Petroleum-based lotions with synthetic fragrances
- Choose: Plant-based oils (coconut, jojoba, argan) or naturally scented lotions
- DIY Simple: Pure coconut oil with a drop of essential oil

- ❖ Makeup:
- Instead of: Conventional makeup with heavy metals and synthetic dyes
- Choose: Mineral makeup, organic brands, or reduce usage
- Priority: Focus on products you use daily (foundation, mascara, lipstick)

- ❖ Sunscreen:
- Instead of: Chemical sunscreens with oxybenzone
- Choose: Mineral sunscreens with zinc oxide or titanium dioxide
- Bonus: Many mineral sunscreens double as makeup primers

Budget-Friendly Transition Strategy

- ❖ Phase 1: Immediate Wins (Under $50)
- Switch to fragrance-free laundry detergent
- Replace antibacterial hand soap with castile soap
- Use coconut oil as moisturizer
- Make your own deodorant or buy one natural version

- ❖ Phase 2: Daily Essentials ($50-150)
- Replace shampoo and conditioner
- Switch to natural deodorant
- Buy mineral sunscreen
- Replace daily makeup items

- ❖ Phase 3: Complete Overhaul ($150+)
- Replace all skincare products
- Switch to organic makeup
- Invest in high-quality, multi-purpose products
- Add air purifier and water filter

- ❖ Money-Saving Tips:
- Many natural ingredients are multi-purpose (coconut oil for moisturizer, makeup remover, and hair treatment)
- Buy in bulk when you find products you love
- Make your own when possible (deodorant, face masks, scrubs)
- Focus on products you use most frequently first

HOUSEHOLD CHEMICALS: CLEANING WITHOUT POISONING

Most commercial household cleaners contain harsh chemicals that linger in your air and on surfaces long after cleaning. You're exposed through inhalation, skin contact, and residues on dishes and surfaces.

The Problem with Conventional Cleaners

- ❖ Common Toxic Ingredients:
- Ammonia: Respiratory irritant, especially dangerous when mixed with bleach
- Chlorine Bleach: Releases toxic chlorine gas, especially when mixed with other chemicals
- Phosphates: Environmental pollutants that can disrupt hormones
- Synthetic Fragrances: VOCs that pollute indoor air for hours
- Antibacterial Agents: Contribute to antibiotic resistance and microbiome disruption
- Volatile Organic Compounds (VOCs): Cause headaches, dizziness, and respiratory issues

The Natural Cleaning Arsenal

- ❖ The Big Four: Your Essential Natural Cleaners
1. White Vinegar: Antimicrobial, cuts grease, removes mineral deposits
2. Baking Soda: Deodorizes, scrubs gently, neutralizes acids
3. Castile Soap: Plant-based cleaner for almost everything
4. Lemon: Natural bleaching, antimicrobial, fresh scent

- ❖ Power Combinations:
- All-Purpose Cleaner: 1 cup water + 1 cup vinegar + 15 drops essential oil
- Scrubbing Paste: Baking soda + small amount of water
- Glass Cleaner: 2 cups water + 1/2 cup vinegar + 1/4 cup rubbing alcohol
- Disinfectant: 1 cup water + 1/2 cup vinegar + 10 drops tea tree oil

Room-by-Room Natural Cleaning Solutions

- ❖ Kitchen:
- Counters: Vinegar solution or castile soap and water
- Oven: Baking soda paste, let sit overnight, scrub and rinse
- Dishwasher: Run empty cycle with 2 cups vinegar in a dishwasher-safe bowl
- Cutting Boards: Scrub with coarse salt and lemon, rinse well

- ❖ Bathroom:
- Toilet: Baking soda + vinegar, let fizz, scrub and flush
- Shower/Tub: Baking soda paste for scrubbing, vinegar for mineral deposits
- Mirrors: Vinegar and water solution with newspaper for streak-free cleaning
- Drains: Monthly flush with baking soda followed by vinegar

- ❖ Living Areas:
- Furniture: Olive oil + lemon juice for wood polish
- Carpets: Baking soda sprinkled, let sit, vacuum for odor removal
- Air Freshening: Simmer cinnamon sticks, orange peels, or use essential oil diffuser
- Dust: Microfiber cloths with water or light castile soap solution

- ❖ Laundry:
- Detergent: Castile soap-based or plant-based commercial brands
- Fabric Softener: 1/2 cup white vinegar in rinse cycle
- Stain Removal: Baking soda paste for most stains, lemon juice for whites
- Whitening: Hydrogen peroxide instead of chlorine bleach

Commercial Natural Product Guidelines

- ❖ If making your own isn't realistic, look for products that are:
- Certified by Third Parties: EWG Verified, Green Seal, or EPA Safer Choice
- Transparent about Ingredients: Full ingredient disclosure
- Plant-Based: Derived from renewable resources
- Concentrated: Less packaging, often more economical
- Fragrance-Free or Naturally Scented: Avoid synthetic fragrances

- ❖ Trusted Brands (always read labels as formulations change):
- Branch Basics (concentrate system)

- Dr. Bronner's (castile soap products)
- Seventh Generation (widely available)
- Ecover (plant-based formulas)
- Method (stylish and effective)

PRACTICAL TOOL: HOME ENVIRONMENTAL AUDIT CHECKLIST

Use this comprehensive checklist to assess and improve your home environment systematically. Rate each area and focus on your lowest scores first.

Air Quality Assessment

Current Status (Rate 1-5: 1=Poor, 5=Excellent):

❖ Ventilation (___/5):
- Open windows daily for fresh air exchange
- Use exhaust fans in kitchen and bathrooms
- Avoid blocking air vents with furniture
- Create cross-ventilation when possible

❖ Indoor Plants (___/5):
- Have air-purifying plants throughout home
- One plant per 100 square feet of space
- Plants are healthy and well-maintained
- Variety of plant types for different pollutants

❖ Chemical Avoidance (___/5):
- No synthetic air fresheners or plug-ins
- No scented candles with synthetic fragrances
- Avoid aerosol sprays and harsh chemicals
- Use natural alternatives for fragrances

❖ Air Purification (___/5):
- Have air purifier with HEPA and carbon filters (if needed)
- Change HVAC filters regularly
- Keep humidity levels between 30-50%
- Address any mold or moisture issues

Priority Action Items:
1. _____
2. _____
3. _____

Water Quality Assessment

Current Status (Rate 1-5):

❖ Drinking Water (___/5):
- Use filtered water for drinking and cooking
- Filter removes chlorine, heavy metals, and other contaminants
- Know what's in your local water supply

- Avoid plastic water bottles

❖ Shower/Bath Water (___/5):
- Have shower filter to remove chlorine
- Bath water is filtered or dechlorinated
- Water temperature is warm, not hot
- Limit bath/shower time to reduce chemical exposure

❖ Hydration Habits (___/5):
- Drink adequate water daily (half body weight in ounces)
- Use glass or stainless steel containers
- Add natural minerals to water
- Monitor hydration status regularly

Priority Action Items:
1. _____
2. _____
3. _____

Personal Care Products Assessment

Current Status (Rate 1-5):

❖ Daily Use Products (___/5):
- Shampoo, conditioner, body wash are natural/organic
- Deodorant is aluminum-free
- Moisturizers are plant-based without synthetic fragrances
- Toothpaste is fluoride-free (if preferred)

❖ Cosmetics and Skincare (___/5):
- Makeup is mineral-based or organic
- Skincare products are free of parabens and phthalates
- Sunscreen is mineral-based (zinc oxide/titanium dioxide)
- Nail products are non-toxic

❖ Men's Grooming (___/5):
- Shaving cream/gel is natural
- Aftershave is alcohol and synthetic fragrance-free
- Hair products are plant-based
- Cologne/fragrance is natural or avoided

Priority Action Items:
1. _____
2. _____
3. _____

Household Cleaning Assessment

Current Status (Rate 1-5):

❖ Cleaning Products (___/5):

- All-purpose cleaners are plant-based or homemade
- Bathroom cleaners are non-toxic
- Kitchen cleaners are food-safe
- Laundry detergent is plant-based and fragrance-free

- ❖ Cleaning Tools (___/5):
- Use microfiber cloths instead of paper towels when possible
- Have glass bottles for homemade cleaners
- Vacuum has HEPA filter
- Cleaning tools are well-maintained

- ❖ Air Freshening (___/5):
- Use natural methods (baking soda, essential oils)
- Avoid synthetic air fresheners completely
- Address odor sources rather than masking
- Open windows for fresh air regularly

Priority Action Items:
1. _____
2. _____
3. _____

Home Environment Assessment

Current Status (Rate 1-5):

- ❖ Furniture and Textiles (___/5):
- Mattress is organic or natural materials
- Furniture is solid wood or metal, not particle board
- Textiles are natural fibers (cotton, linen, wool)
- Carpets are natural fiber or hard flooring

- ❖ Kitchen Safety (___/5):
- Cookware is stainless steel, cast iron, or ceramic
- Food storage is glass or stainless steel
- Avoid heating food in plastic containers
- Use parchment paper instead of plastic wrap

- ❖ Bedroom Environment (___/5):
- Electronics are minimal or removed
- Bedding is organic cotton or natural fibers
- Room has good ventilation
- Sleep environment is cool, dark, and quiet

- ❖ Home Office (___/5):
- Good ventilation and natural light
- Plants for air purification
- Ergonomic setup to reduce physical stress
- Regular breaks and movement

Priority Action Items:
1. _____
2. _____
3. _____

Overall Assessment Summary

Total Score: ___/100

❖ Score Interpretation:
- 80-100: Excellent environmental health practices
- 60-79: Good foundation with room for targeted improvements
- 40-59: Moderate environmental health, several areas need attention
- 20-39: High toxic load, systematic changes recommended
- Below 20: Very high toxic exposure, immediate action needed

Top 3 Priority Areas (focus here first):
1. _____
2. _____
3. _____

30-Day Action Plan

❖ Week 1: Focus on highest-impact, lowest-cost changes
- Replace air fresheners with essential oils or remove completely
- Switch to natural cleaning products or make your own
- Add houseplants to main living areas
- Start drinking filtered water

❖ Week 2: Personal care product swaps
- Replace daily-use products (shampoo, deodorant, lotion)
- Switch to natural toothpaste
- Choose mineral sunscreen
- Reduce or eliminate synthetic fragrances

❖ Week 3: Kitchen and food safety
- Replace plastic food storage with glass
- Check cookware for non-stick coatings
- Switch to natural dish soap
- Filter shower water if possible

❖ Week 4: Bedroom optimization
- Remove unnecessary electronics
- Switch to organic bedding if possible
- Add bedroom plants
- Improve ventilation

Maintenance Schedule

❖ Daily:
- Open windows for fresh air (weather permitting)

- Use natural cleaning products
- Drink filtered water
- Check ingredient labels on new products

❖ Weekly:
- Water houseplants and check their health
- Clean with natural products
- Wash bedding in natural detergent
- Assess any new products before purchase

❖ Monthly:
- Replace water filters
- Deep clean with natural products
- Evaluate and replace any products that aren't working
- Add new plants or natural improvements

❖ Seasonally:
- Deep clean air vents and replace HVAC filters
- Assess overall air quality and make improvements
- Update cleaning supplies and natural products
- Evaluate progress and set new goals

Chapter 10 Key Takeaways

❖ What You Learned:
- Your home environment significantly impacts your inflammatory burden
- Small, strategic changes can dramatically reduce your daily toxic load
- Natural alternatives exist for virtually every household product
- Air and water quality are foundational to environmental health
- Progress matters more than perfection

❖ What You Can Do Right Now:
- Complete the Home Environmental Audit Checklist
- Remove one source of synthetic fragrance from your home
- Open windows for 10 minutes to improve air quality
- Switch to one natural personal care product
- Start reading ingredient labels before purchasing

Breakfast Recipes

Black Garlic & Wild Salmon

Servings: 2 Prep Time: 10 minutes

Cook Time: 25 minutes

For the teff polenta:

½ cup teff grain

2 cups filtered water

1 tsp extra virgin olive oil

Pinch of Himalayan salt

For the salmon:

2 wild salmon fillets (about 4–5 oz each)

1 tbsp black garlic paste (or 4 cloves mashed)

1 tsp lemon juice

1 tsp grated fresh turmeric (or ¼ tsp powder)

1 tsp avocado oil

For the dandelion greens:

2 cups chopped dandelion greens

1 garlic clove (optional: aged or black garlic)

1 tsp olive oil

1 tsp apple cider vinegar

1. Cook the Teff Polenta

Rinse teff briefly in warm water.

In a saucepan, bring 2 cups water to boil.

Stir in teff, reduce to low heat, and simmer 20–22 minutes, stirring occasionally until creamy.

Stir in olive oil and salt at the end. Cover and set aside.

2. Prepare the Salmon

Preheat oven to 375°F (190°C).

Rub salmon with black garlic paste, turmeric, lemon juice, and a bit of avocado oil.

Place in parchment-lined tray and bake for 10–12 minutes, until flaky.

3. Sauté Dandelion Greens

Heat olive oil in a pan over medium.

Add garlic (if using), sauté for 30 seconds.

Add chopped dandelion greens, cook for 2–3 minutes, until just wilted.

Finish with apple cider vinegar.

To Serve:

Spoon teff polenta onto plates.

Top with baked salmon.

Serve with warm dandelion greens on the side.

Optional: Garnish with fresh parsley or a few crushed walnuts.

Artichoke & Turmeric-Fennel Chickpea Cakes

Servings: 3 (makes \6 cakes) Prep Time: 15 minutes

Cook Time: 15 minutes

For the Chickpea Cakes:

1½ cups cooked chickpeas (or canned, rinsed)

1 cup cooked artichoke hearts (frozen or canned in water)

1 tsp ground turmeric

1 tsp ground fennel seeds

1 small garlic clove (optional: aged or roasted)

2 tbsp finely chopped parsley

2 tbsp ground flaxseed

1 tbsp olive oil (for pan)

Pinch sea salt

For the Lemon-Tahini Sauce:

3 tbsp tahini

Juice of 1 lemon

2–3 tbsp filtered water (to thin)

Pinch cumin or black seed powder (optional)

Pinch sea salt

1. Make the Chickpea Cakes

In a food processor, combine chickpeas, artichokes, turmeric, fennel, garlic, parsley, flaxseed, and salt.

Pulse until a coarse dough forms.

Shape into 6 small patties using damp hands.

2. Heat olive oil in a non-stick or ceramic skillet over medium.

Cook patties 3–4 minutes per side until golden and firm.

3. In a bowl, whisk tahini, lemon juice, water, salt, and cumin/black seed until smooth.

To Serve

Drizzle cakes with lemon-tahini sauce.

Optional sides: bitter greens, cucumber ribbons, or a beet salad.

Sardine-Nori Lettuce Wraps with Avocado

Servings: 2 (makes \4–6 wraps)

Prep Time: 15 minutes

For the wraps:

1 can wild sardines in olive oil or water (boneless optional)

4–6 large romaine or butter lettuce leaves

2 nori sheets, cut into quarters

½ ripe avocado, sliced

1 cup shredded purple cabbage

1 small carrot, grated (optional)

1 tsp sesame seeds (optional)

For the ginger-miso dressing:

1 tbsp white miso (fermented, unpasteurized if possible)

1 tsp fresh grated ginger

1 tbsp lemon or lime juice

1 tsp avocado oil

1–2 tsp warm water (to thin)

1. In a small bowl, whisk miso, ginger, citrus juice, oil, and water until smooth.

2. Assemble Wraps

Lay out lettuce leaves.

Place a piece of nori on each leaf.

Top with shredded cabbage, a sardine (or half), avocado slice, and optional carrot.

Drizzle lightly with ginger-miso dressing.

Sprinkle sesame seeds if using.

3. Fold and eat as hand wraps or roll burrito-style.

Tips

For a warm element, lightly toast nori in a dry pan for 10 seconds until crisp.

Use raw fermented miso for optimal probiotic benefit.

Add a few microgreens or sprouts for an extra anti-inflammatory boost.

Black Lentil & Pomegranate Molasses Bowl

Servings: 2 Prep Time: 10 minutes

Cook Time: 25 minutes

¾ cup dry black lentils (or 1½ cups cooked)

2 large carrots, sliced

1 tbsp olive oil (divided)

1 tbsp pomegranate molasses

2 tbsp chopped fresh mint

½ tsp ground cumin

Pinch of sea salt

Optional garnish: pomegranate seeds

1. Cook Lentils

Rinse lentils and add to a saucepan with 2 cups water.

Bring to boil, reduce heat, simmer uncovered for 18–20 minutes until tender but not mushy.

Drain and set aside.

2. Roast Carrots

Preheat oven to 400°F (200°C).

Toss sliced carrots with ½ tbsp olive oil, cumin, and salt.

Roast on a lined tray for 20–25 minutes, turning once, until golden and soft.

3. Assemble the Bowl

In a bowl, combine lentils, roasted carrots, chopped mint, and remaining olive oil.

Drizzle with pomegranate molasses and gently toss.

To Serve

Divide into bowls.

Top with extra mint and optional pomegranate seeds for texture and color.

Serve warm or at room temperature.

Sunchoke & Leek Soup with Parsley Oil

Servings: 3–4 Prep Time: 10 minutes

Cook Time: 25 minutes

For the soup:

1 tbsp cold-pressed olive oil

2 medium leeks (white/light green parts only), sliced

2 cups sunchokes, scrubbed & diced

2 cloves garlic (aged or fresh), minced

3½ cups filtered vegetable broth

Pinch sea salt

For the parsley oil:

½ cup flat-leaf parsley

3 tbsp extra virgin olive oil

½ small garlic clove

Pinch lemon zest

For the gremolata:

2 tbsp raw pumpkin seeds, chopped

1 tbsp parsley, finely chopped

Zest of ½ lemon

1. Sauté the Base

In a soup pot, warm olive oil over medium heat.

Add leeks and cook 4–5 minutes until soft, not browned.

Add garlic and diced sunchokes, stir 2 minutes.

2. Simmer the Soup

Add vegetable broth and a pinch of salt.

Bring to a boil, reduce heat, and simmer 15–18 minutes, until sunchokes are very tender.

3. Blend Until Creamy

Use an immersion blender or high-speed blender to puree until smooth.

Taste and adjust seasoning.

4. Blend parsley, olive oil, garlic, and lemon zest until smooth and bright green.

5. Mix chopped pumpkin seeds, parsley, and lemon zest in a bowl.

To Serve

Ladle soup into bowls.

Drizzle with parsley oil and sprinkle with gremolata.

Optional: Add a few drops of pumpkin seed oil for extra richness.

Okra, Quinoa & Fermented Lemon Stew

Servings: 3 Prep Time: 10 minutes

Cook Time: 25 minutes

1 tbsp cold-pressed olive oil

1 small onion, chopped

1 tsp fenugreek seeds

1 tsp ground coriander

1½ cups chopped fresh okra (or frozen, thawed)

½ cup white or red quinoa, rinsed

¼ preserved/fermented lemon, finely chopped (peel only)

3 cups filtered water or vegetable broth

2 tbsp chopped fresh cilantro (optional)

Pinch sea salt

1. Toast Spices & Aromatics

In a pot, heat olive oil on medium.

Add onion, fenugreek seeds, and coriander.

Sauté for 3–4 minutes, stirring, until fragrant and translucent.

2. Simmer the Stew

Add okra, quinoa, and water/broth.

Bring to a boil, then reduce to low heat.

Simmer 15–18 minutes, until quinoa is cooked and okra is soft.

3. Add Fermented Lemon

Stir in chopped preserved lemon.

Simmer 2–3 minutes more to infuse flavor.

Add sea salt to taste.

To Serve

Ladle into bowls.

Garnish with fresh cilantro or microgreens if desired.

Pair with a few slices of anti-inflammatory cassava or seed flatbread.

Smoked Mackerel, Kohlrabi & Beet Slaw

Servings: 2

Prep Time: 15 minutes

1 small raw beet, peeled and grated

1 small kohlrabi, peeled and grated or julienned

1 hot-smoked wild mackerel fillet (boneless, skin removed)

1 tbsp prepared horseradish (no sugar/additives)

1½ tbsp apple cider vinegar

1 tbsp cold-pressed flaxseed or extra virgin olive oil

Pinch sea salt

1 tsp chopped fresh dill or parsley (optional)

1. Make the Slaw Base

In a bowl, combine grated beet and kohlrabi.

Toss gently with a pinch of salt to soften slightly.

2. Prepare the Dressing

In a small bowl, whisk together horseradish, vinegar, and oil.

Taste and adjust with a bit more vinegar if needed.

3. Assemble the Bowl

Gently flake the smoked mackerel over the slaw.

Drizzle with the horseradish-vinegar dressing.

Sprinkle with fresh herbs if using.

To Serve

Serve immediately as a light meal or hearty appetizer.

Optional: Add a handful of arugula or watercress for an extra anti-inflammatory boost.

Shiitake Mushroom & Bok Choy Hotpot

Servings: 2–3 Prep Time: 10 minutes

Cook Time: 20 minutes

- 1 tbsp cold-pressed sesame or olive oil
- 1 cup fresh shiitake mushrooms (or rehydrated dried), sliced
- 2 cups chopped bok choy (both stems and leaves)
- 4 black garlic cloves (or 1 tbsp paste), mashed
- 3 cups filtered vegetable broth
- 1 star anise pod
- 1-inch piece of fresh ginger, sliced thin
- 1 tbsp coconut aminos or fermented tamari (gluten-free, low-sodium)
- Optional: ½ tsp crushed red pepper or chili flakes
- Optional garnish: chopped cilantro or green onions

1. Sauté Aromatics

Heat oil in a pot over medium heat.

Add ginger and black garlic. Sauté 2 minutes until fragrant.

Add sliced shiitake and stir for 3–4 minutes, until softened slightly.

2. Simmer Broth

Pour in broth. Add star anise and coconut aminos.

Bring to a low boil, then reduce heat and simmer uncovered for 10 minutes.

3. Add bok choy and simmer for 3–5 minutes, until just tender but still vibrant.

To Serve

Remove star anise pod.

Ladle hotpot into bowls.

Garnish with cilantro, green onion, or a drizzle of sesame oil (optional).

Green Papaya & Avocado Salad

Servings: 2

Prep Time: 10 minutes

1 cup shredded green (unripe) papaya

½ ripe avocado, diced

2 tbsp raw macadamia nuts, roughly chopped

¼ cup fresh cilantro or Thai basil (optional)

For the vinaigrette:

1 tbsp freshly squeezed lime juice

1 tsp grated fresh ginger

1 tsp extra virgin olive oil or macadamia oil

Pinch of sea salt

1. In a small bowl, whisk lime juice, grated ginger, oil, and salt.

2. Assemble the Salad

In a mixing bowl, combine shredded green papaya, diced avocado, and herbs (if using).

Drizzle with vinaigrette and toss gently to coat.

3. Top and Serve

Sprinkle with chopped macadamia nuts just before serving for crunch.

Serve immediately as a refreshing side or light anti-inflammatory main.

Tips

To shred green papaya: peel it, remove seeds, and use a julienne slicer or box grater.

For added anti-inflammatory benefit, top with a small handful of watercress or sprouts.

Chaga-Infused Wild Rice Pilaf

Servings: 3 Prep Time: 10 minutes

Cook Time: 40 minutes

¾ cup wild rice

2 cups chaga tea (see instructions below)

¼ cup dried unsweetened cranberries

¼ cup raw hazelnuts, roughly chopped

1 tbsp olive oil or avocado oil

1½ tsp chopped fresh or dried tarragon

Pinch sea salt

To Make Chaga Tea

Simmer 1 tbsp powdered or chunked chaga mushroom in 2½ cups water for 15–20 minutes.

Strain and use 2 cups of the tea for cooking rice.

Make extra and drink the rest — it's great for inflammation.

1. Cook the Wild Rice

Rinse wild rice thoroughly.

In a pot, combine rice and 2 cups chaga tea.

Bring to a boil, then reduce heat, cover, and simmer for 35–40 minutes, or until rice is tender and liquid is absorbed.

Let sit covered for 5 minutes.

2. While rice cooks, dry-toast hazelnuts in a skillet over medium heat for 3–4 minutes, until aromatic. Set aside.

3. Fluff rice with a fork. Stir in cranberries, toasted hazelnuts, tarragon, olive oil, and a pinch of salt.

To Serve

Serve warm as a main or side.

Optional: top with a few fresh microgreens or drizzle of cold-pressed flax oil.

Golden Cauliflower & Broccoli Stir-Fry

Servings: 2 Prep Time: 10 minutes

Cook Time: 10 minutes

For the stir-fry:

1 cup broccoli florets

1 cup cauliflower florets

1 tsp ground turmeric

1 tbsp cold-pressed avocado or olive oil

Pinch of sea salt

Squeeze of lemon (to finish)

For the basil-pistachio pesto:

½ cup fresh basil leaves

2 tbsp raw pistachios

1 small garlic clove

1 tbsp lemon juice

2 tbsp extra virgin olive oil

1–2 tsp water (to thin, as needed)

Pinch of sea salt

1. Make the Pesto

In a small blender or food processor, blend basil, pistachios, garlic, lemon juice, and olive oil until smooth.

Add a splash of water if needed to loosen texture. Set aside.

2. Sauté the Veggies

Heat oil in a large skillet or wok over medium heat.

Add broccoli and cauliflower. Stir-fry for 2 minutes.

Sprinkle turmeric evenly over the vegetables. Stir again.

Add a splash of water (1–2 tbsp), cover, and steam for 4–5 minutes until just tender but still vibrant.

3. Finish & Assemble

Remove lid, season lightly with salt.

Turn off heat, squeeze fresh lemon over vegetables.

Spoon pesto generously over the warm veggies.

To Serve

Serve warm as a main or side.

Optionally top with a few extra chopped pistachios or fresh basil ribbons.

Buckwheat-Kale Pancakes

Servings: 2 (makes \6 small pancakes) Prep Time: 15 minutes (plus soak/ferment time)

Cook Time: 10 minutes

For the pancakes:

½ cup buckwheat flour

½ tsp baking soda (aluminum-free)

½ cup finely chopped kale (massaged or lightly steamed)

1 flax egg (1 tbsp ground flax + 3 tbsp water, rested 5 min)

⅓ cup filtered water

1 tbsp olive oil (plus more for cooking)

Pinch sea salt

For the fermented cashew ricotta:

½ cup raw cashews (soaked 4–6 hrs, drained)

2 tbsp water

½ tsp lemon juice

½ tsp unpasteurized miso or a probiotic capsule

Pinch sea salt

1. Make the Cashew Ricotta (Ferment First)

Blend soaked cashews, lemon, water, and salt until smooth.

Stir in miso or probiotic powder if fermenting.

Transfer to a clean glass jar, cover loosely, and ferment at room temp for 12–24 hours (optional but recommended).

Store in fridge up to 5 days.

2. Prepare the Pancake Batter

In a bowl, whisk together buckwheat flour, baking soda, and salt.

Stir in flax egg, water, and olive oil.

Fold in chopped kale. Let batter rest 5 minutes.

3. Cook the Pancakes

Heat a ceramic or cast-iron skillet over medium.

Lightly grease with olive oil.

Pour small rounds of batter into skillet; cook 2–3 minutes per side, until golden and firm.

To Serve

Top warm pancakes with a dollop of fermented cashew ricotta.

Sprinkle generously with sumac.

Charred Eggplant, Lentil & Za'atar-Stuffed Collard Wraps

Servings: 2 (makes 4 wraps) Prep Time: 15 minutes

Cook Time: 15–20 minutes

For the filling:

- 1 small eggplant (keep skin on), sliced
- ¾ cup cooked green or black lentils
- 1 tbsp za'atar (unsalted, no fillers)
- 1 tbsp cold-pressed olive oil
- Pinch of sea salt

For the wraps:

- 4 large collard green leaves (stems trimmed flat)
- Juice of ½ lemon
- Optional: 1 tsp tahini or 1 tbsp diced cucumber for topping

1. Char the Eggplant

Brush eggplant slices lightly with olive oil.

Grill, broil, or pan-sear over high heat for 3–4 minutes per side, until soft and lightly charred.

Let cool slightly, then dice.

2. Mix the Filling

Combine chopped eggplant, lentils, za'atar, a drizzle of olive oil, and a pinch of sea salt.

Mix well and set aside.

3. Prep the Collard Wraps

Bring a wide pot of water to a boil.

Blanch collard leaves for 30–45 seconds to soften.

Transfer to an ice bath or cool under running water, then pat dry.

4. Assemble the Wraps

Lay a collard leaf flat.

Spoon in the eggplant-lentil filling.

Add a drizzle of lemon juice and optional tahini or cucumber.

Fold in sides and roll tightly like a burrito.

Optional garnish: sprinkle extra za'atar on top, or serve with a side of probiotic kraut or fermented radishes.

Golden Beet, Arugula & Hemp Heart Salad

Servings: 2 Prep Time: 10 minutes

Cook Time: 20 minutes (for beets)

For the salad:

2 small golden beets, peeled and sliced into wedges

2 cups fresh arugula

2 tbsp hemp hearts

Optional: a few thinly sliced cucumber rounds or microgreens

For the saffron-honey vinaigrette:

1 tbsp warm water

5–6 saffron threads

1 tsp raw honey (or bee-free fermented honey alt)

1½ tbsp fresh lemon juice

1½ tbsp extra virgin olive oil

Pinch of sea salt

1. Cook the Beets

Steam or boil beet wedges until just tender, 15–20 minutes.

Let cool to room temperature (can chill slightly if desired).

2. Make the Vinaigrette

Steep saffron threads in warm water for 5 minutes.

Whisk in honey, lemon juice, olive oil, and salt until emulsified.

3. Assemble the Salad

In a large bowl, toss arugula with cooled beets.

Drizzle with saffron-honey vinaigrette.

Sprinkle hemp hearts on top.

Add cucumber or microgreens if using.

Optional pairing: a spoonful of cultured coconut yogurt or sprouted seed crackers on the side.

Lotus Root & Adzuki Bean Stir-Fry

Servings: 2 Prep Time: 10 minutes (beans pre-cooked or soaked)

Cook Time: 20 minutes

- 1 cup thinly sliced lotus root (peeled)
- ¾ cup cooked adzuki beans (or canned, drained & rinsed)
- 1 tbsp cold-pressed coconut oil
- 1½ tsp freshly grated turmeric (or ½ tsp ground)
- 1 cup light coconut milk
- ½ cup filtered water or veggie broth
- 1 tsp grated fresh ginger
- 1 tsp coconut aminos (optional)
- Pinch sea salt
- Garnish: chopped fresh cilantro or Thai basil

1. Sauté Aromatics

Heat coconut oil in a sauté pan over medium heat.

Add ginger and turmeric. Stir for 30–60 seconds until fragrant.

2. Add Lotus Root & Beans

Add sliced lotus root and stir-fry for 2–3 minutes.

Stir in adzuki beans and cook another 2 minutes.

3. Simmer in Broth

Pour in coconut milk and water.

Add a pinch of salt and optional coconut aminos.

Bring to a low simmer and cook 8–10 minutes, until lotus root is tender-crisp and broth is slightly thickened.

To Serve

Spoon into shallow bowls.

Garnish with fresh cilantro or Thai basil.

Optional: Serve over steamed red rice, fonio, or just enjoy as a light stew.

Lunch and Dinner Options

Turmeric-Infused Lentil Soup

Servings: 3 Prep Time: 10 minutes

Cook Time: 20 minutes

¾ cup red lentils (rinsed)

1½ cups water or low-sodium vegetable broth

½ cup full-fat coconut milk

1½ tsp freshly grated turmeric (or ¾ tsp ground)

1 tsp black mustard seeds

½ tsp ground cumin

1 clove garlic, minced

1 tbsp finely chopped ginger

1 tbsp cold-pressed coconut oil

Pinch of sea salt

Optional: chopped fresh coriander for garnish

1. Bloom the Spices

In a pot, heat coconut oil on medium.

Add mustard seeds and let them pop (about 30 seconds).

Stir in ginger, garlic, turmeric, and cumin. Sauté for 1 minute until fragrant.

2. Simmer the Soup

Add lentils and water or broth. Bring to a boil.

Reduce heat and simmer 15–18 minutes, until lentils are soft.

3. Finish with Coconut Milk

Stir in coconut milk and simmer gently for 2–3 minutes.

Add sea salt to taste.

To Serve:

Serve warm, optionally garnished with coriander or a squeeze of lime.

Pairs beautifully with sautéed kale, collard greens, or a spoon of fermented carrot slaw.

Grilled Sardines with Stewed Tomatoes, Olives & Fennel over Millet

Servings: 2 Prep Time: 10 minutes

Cook Time: 25 minutes

For the sardines:

4 fresh sardines, cleaned

1 tbsp olive oil

½ tsp lemon zest

Pinch sea salt

For the stewed tomato-olive-fennel mix:

1 cup chopped tomatoes (fresh or low-sodium canned)

½ cup thinly sliced fennel bulb

¼ cup pitted green or black olives, halved

1 tsp olive oil

1 small garlic clove, minced

½ tsp dried oregano or thyme

For the millet:

½ cup millet

1½ cups water

Pinch salt

1. Cook the Millet

Rinse millet thoroughly.

Add to a pot with water and salt.

Bring to a boil, reduce heat, cover, and simmer 15–18 minutes until fluffy. Set aside.

2. Make the Stewed Tomatoes

In a skillet, heat 1 tsp olive oil over medium.

Add garlic and fennel, sauté 2–3 minutes.

Add tomatoes, olives, herbs, and simmer 10–12 minutes, until soft and slightly reduced.

3. Grill the Sardines

Rub sardines with olive oil, lemon zest, and a pinch of salt.

Grill (or pan-sear) on medium-high heat for 2–3 minutes per side until skin is crisp and flesh opaque.

To Serve:

Plate a bed of millet.

Spoon tomato-fennel-olive stew over it.

Top with grilled sardines.

Optional: garnish with fresh fennel fronds or parsley.

Miso-Braised Turnips & Shiitake Mushrooms

Servings: 2 Prep Time: 10 minutes

Cook Time: 25 minutes

For the rice:

½ cup black rice

1 cup water

Pinch sea salt

For the miso-braised vegetables:

1 cup peeled, cubed turnips

1 cup sliced fresh shiitake mushrooms

1 tbsp mellow white or brown miso

½ cup warm water

1 tsp grated fresh ginger

1 tsp toasted sesame oil (optional)

1 tsp rice vinegar (unseasoned)

1 tsp coconut aminos (optional for umami)

1. Roast the Sweet Potatoes & Chickpeas

Preheat oven to 400°F (200°C).

Toss cubed sweet potatoes and chickpeas with olive oil, cumin, paprika, and a pinch of salt.

Spread on a baking sheet and roast for 20–25 minutes, flipping halfway, until golden and crisp on edges.

2. While roasting, sauté kale in a splash of water or ½ tsp olive oil over medium heat for **2–3 minutes**, just until wilted. Set aside.

3. Whisk tahini, lemon juice, cumin, salt, and water until smooth and pourable.

To Serve

In bowls, layer roasted sweet potatoes, chickpeas, and kale.

Drizzle generously with cumin-tahini sauce.

Optional: top with sesame seeds, sumac, or hemp hearts.

Wild-Caught Salmon with Roasted Purple Cauliflower

Servings: 2 Prep Time: 10 minutes

Cook Time: 20 minutes

For the salmon:

2 wild-caught salmon fillets (\4–5 oz each)

1 tsp lemon zest

1 tsp olive oil

Pinch sea salt

For the roasted cauliflower:

2 cups purple cauliflower florets

1 tbsp olive oil

½ tsp ground turmeric

Pinch sea salt

For the gremolata:

1 clove garlic (raw or roasted, finely minced)

2 tbsp finely chopped parsley

Zest of ½ lemon

1 tsp olive oil

1. Roast the Cauliflower

Preheat oven to 400°F (200°C).

Toss cauliflower with olive oil, turmeric, and salt.

Spread on a baking sheet and roast for 18–20 minutes, flipping once, until tender and lightly browned.

2. Prepare the Salmon

Rub salmon with olive oil, lemon zest, and a pinch of salt.

Grill or pan-sear over medium heat for 3–4 minutes per side, or bake in the oven for **10–12 minutes**, until just opaque.

3. Make the Gremolata

Mix garlic, parsley, lemon zest, and olive oil in a small bowl.

Let sit 5 minutes for flavors to meld.

To Serve

Plate roasted purple cauliflower alongside salmon.

Spoon gremolata over the salmon just before serving.

Optional: garnish with microgreens or crushed walnuts for extra anti-inflammatory boost.

Stuffed Collard Wraps with Quinoa

Servings: 2 (4–6 wraps) Prep Time: 15 minutes

Cook Time: 15 minutes

For the wraps:

4 large collard green leaves

½ cup cooked quinoa

1 medium carrot, grated

2 tbsp chopped fresh cilantro

2 tbsp thinly sliced red cabbage (optional)

For the ginger-lime dressing:

1½ tbsp fresh lime juice

1 tsp grated fresh ginger

1 tbsp extra virgin olive oil or avocado oil

½ tsp raw honey (optional; omit if low-sugar)

Pinch sea salt

1. Blanch the Collard Leaves

Trim the thick bottom stem of each leaf to make them more pliable.

Bring a wide pan of water to a gentle boil.

Blanch leaves for 30 seconds, then plunge into cold water. Pat dry.

2. Prepare the Filling

In a bowl, mix cooked quinoa, grated carrot, chopped cilantro, and cabbage (if using).

Whisk dressing ingredients together in a small bowl.

Pour over quinoa mixture and toss to combine.

3. Assemble the Wraps

Lay a collard leaf flat, dark side down.

Spoon 2–3 tbsp of filling near the base.

Fold in sides, then roll tightly like a burrito.

To Serve

Slice each wrap in half diagonally.

Serve chilled or at room temp with extra ginger-lime drizzle or avocado slices.

Carrot-Ginger Soup with Coconut & Red Lentils

Servings: 3 Prep Time: 10 minutes

Cook Time: 20 minutes

- 1 cup carrots, sliced
- ½ cup red lentils (rinsed)
- 2 cups filtered water or low-sodium veg broth
- ½ cup full-fat coconut milk
- 1 tbsp fresh ginger, grated
- 1 small garlic clove (optional)
- 1 tbsp olive or coconut oil
- Sea salt to taste
- Handful fresh mint leaves, chopped (for topping)

1. Sauté Aromatics

In a pot, heat oil over medium.

Add ginger and garlic (if using), sauté 1 minute until fragrant.

2. Simmer the Base

Add carrots, lentils, and water/broth.

Bring to a boil, then reduce heat.

Simmer 15–18 minutes, until carrots and lentils are soft.

3. Blend & Finish

Stir in coconut milk.

Blend until smooth using an immersion blender or high-speed blender.

Add salt to taste.

To Serve

Pour into bowls, top with chopped fresh mint.

Optional: drizzle of flaxseed or MCT oil for an extra anti-inflammatory boost.

Buckwheat Noodles with Charred Broccoli

Servings: 2 Prep Time: 10 minutes

Cook Time: 15 minutes

For the bowl:

4 oz (about 120g) 100% buckwheat soba noodles

2 cups broccoli florets

1 sheet nori, torn or sliced into strips

1 tsp toasted sesame seeds (optional)

1 tsp olive or avocado oil

For the sesame-miso dressing:

1 tbsp white or yellow miso paste

1 tbsp tahini

1 tbsp warm water

1 tsp toasted sesame oil

½ tsp grated ginger

1 tsp lemon juice

1. Char the Broccoli

Heat oil in a skillet over medium-high.

Add broccoli florets and cook 5–6 minutes, turning occasionally, until slightly charred but still crisp. Set aside.

2. Cook the Noodles

Boil soba noodles according to package (usually 5–6 minutes).

Rinse under cold water to stop cooking. Drain well.

3. In a bowl, whisk miso, tahini, lemon juice, sesame oil, ginger, and warm water until smooth.

4. Assemble

Toss noodles with dressing.

Top with charred broccoli and shredded nori.

Garnish with sesame seeds if desired.

To Serve

Serve chilled or at room temperature.

Optional: Add a squeeze of lime or sprinkle of finely chopped scallions or microgreens for extra brightness.

Roasted Brussels Sprouts & Grapes

Servings: 2 Prep Time: 10 minutes

Cook Time: 25 minutes

For the bowl:

1 cup cooked freekeh

1 cup halved Brussels sprouts

½ cup red grapes (halved)

1 tbsp olive oil

Pinch sea salt

For the balsamic reduction:

¼ cup high-quality aged balsamic vinegar (no added sugar)

1. Cook the Freekeh

In a pot, combine ½ cup dry freekeh with 1½ cups water and a pinch of salt.

Bring to a boil, then simmer covered for 20 minutes or until tender.

Fluff and set aside.

2. Roast Brussels Sprouts & Grapes

Preheat oven to 400°F (200°C).

Toss sprouts and grapes with olive oil and a pinch of salt.

Spread on a baking sheet and roast for 18–20 minutes, until sprouts are golden and grapes begin to blister.

3. In a small pan, simmer balsamic vinegar over low heat 6–8 minutes, until thickened and syrupy. Watch closely to avoid burning.

To Serve

Plate freekeh as the base.

Top with roasted sprouts and grapes.

Drizzle generously with balsamic reduction.

Optional: sprinkle of crushed walnuts or microgreens.

Eggplant & Tomato Tagine with Chickpeas

Servings: 2 Prep Time: 10 minutes

Cook Time: 25 minutes

- 1 medium eggplant, cubed (with skin)
- 1 cup canned diced tomatoes (no added salt/sugar)
- 1 cup cooked chickpeas (or 1 can, rinsed)
- 1 small red onion, chopped
- 1 clove garlic, minced
- 1 tsp ground cinnamon
- ½ tsp ground cumin
- 2 tbsp olive oil
- ¼ cup water or veggie broth
- Sea salt to taste
- 2 tbsp chopped fresh parsley (for garnish)

1. Sauté the Aromatics

Heat olive oil in a deep skillet or tagine pot over medium.

Add onion and garlic, sauté for 2–3 minutes until translucent.

Stir in cinnamon and cumin.

2. Simmer the Tagine

Add eggplant cubes, diced tomatoes, chickpeas, and water/broth.

Bring to a simmer, then reduce heat and cover.

Cook for 18–20 minutes, stirring occasionally, until eggplant is soft and sauce thickens slightly.

Add salt to taste.

3. Finish & Serve

Remove from heat and stir in fresh parsley.

Let sit 2 minutes to meld flavors.

To Serve

Serve warm, optionally over millet, cauliflower rice, or quinoa.

Garnish with extra parsley, lemon zest, or a drizzle of cold-pressed flaxseed oil.

Golden Beet & Arugula Salad with Hemp Seeds

Servings: 2 Prep Time: 10 minutes

Cook Time: 25 minutes (roasting beets)

For the salad:

2 small golden beets

2 cups baby arugula

2 tbsp hemp seeds

Optional: thin slices of fennel or radish (for crunch)

For the vinaigrette:

2 tbsp pomegranate juice (100% pure)

1 tbsp extra virgin olive oil

½ tsp lemon juice or apple cider vinegar

Pinch of sea salt

Optional: ¼ tsp finely grated ginger or shallot

1. Roast the Beets

Preheat oven to 400°F (200°C).

Scrub beets, wrap in foil or place in a covered dish, and roast for **25–30 minutes** or until fork-tender.

Cool slightly, then peel and slice into rounds or wedges.

2. Prepare the Vinaigrette

Whisk together pomegranate juice, olive oil, lemon juice, salt, and ginger (if using).

Let sit 5–10 minutes to meld flavors.

3. Assemble the Salad

In a bowl, combine arugula and roasted beets.

Drizzle with vinaigrette and toss gently.

Top with hemp seeds (and fennel or radish if using).

Optional: Add microgreens or a sprinkle of sumac for extra polyphenols.

Amaranth-Crusted Tempeh with Braised Cabbage

Servings: 2 Prep Time: 15 minutes

Cook Time: 20 minutes

For the tempeh:

1 block (about 200g) tempeh, sliced into ½-inch strips

¼ cup amaranth seeds (raw, uncooked)

1 tbsp ground flax + 2½ tbsp water (flax egg)

½ tsp smoked paprika or turmeric

1 tsp olive oil (for pan-frying)

For the braised cabbage:

2 cups shredded red or green cabbage

1 tsp apple cider vinegar

1 tsp olive oil

¼ cup water

Pinch of sea salt

For the horseradish cream:

2 tbsp unsweetened coconut yogurt (or cashew yogurt)

½–1 tsp freshly grated horseradish

1. Prepare the Flax Egg & Crust

Mix flax and water, let sit 5 minutes.

Spread raw amaranth seeds on a plate and mix with paprika or turmeric.

2. Dip each tempeh slice in flax mixture, then press into amaranth to coat both sides.

3. Pan-Fry the Tempeh

Heat 1 tsp oil in a skillet over medium.

Cook tempeh strips for 3–4 minutes per side, until golden and crispy. Set aside.

4. Braise the Cabbage

In a separate pan, heat olive oil, add cabbage, and sauté briefly.

Add vinegar, water, and salt.

Cover and cook on low for 8–10 minutes, until soft but vibrant.

5. Stir together yogurt, horseradish, lemon juice, and salt.

To Serve

Plate the braised cabbage, top with crispy amaranth-crusted tempeh.

Drizzle or dollop with horseradish cream.

Optional: Garnish with parsley or microgreens.

Sunchoke & Asparagus Stir-Fry with Cumin

Servings: 2 Prep Time: 10 minutes

Cook Time: 12 minutes

1 cup thinly sliced sunchokes (scrubbed, skin-on)

1 cup asparagus, trimmed and cut into 2-inch pieces

1 garlic clove, minced

½ tsp ground cumin

1 tbsp cold-pressed avocado oil (or olive oil)

2 tbsp raw pumpkin seeds (pepitas)

Sea salt to taste

Optional: pinch of crushed coriander seed or lemon zest

1. In a dry skillet, toast pumpkin seeds over medium heat for 2–3 minutes, stirring often until they pop and lightly brown. Remove and set aside.

2. Sauté the Sunchokes

Add oil to the same pan and heat over medium.

Add sliced sunchokes and a pinch of salt. Sauté for 5–6 minutes, stirring occasionally, until golden and slightly soft.

3. Add Asparagus & Aromatics

Add asparagus, garlic, and cumin (plus coriander/lemon zest if using).

Stir-fry for another 4–5 minutes, until asparagus is just tender and bright green. Adjust salt as needed.

4. Finish & Serve

Stir in toasted pumpkin seeds.

Remove from heat and let sit 1 minute for flavors to meld.

To Serve

Serve warm as a side or over quinoa, teff, or sprouted lentils for a light meal.

Optional drizzle: flax oil or tahini-lemon sauce.

Thai Coconut Soup with Lemongrass, Mushrooms, Bok Choy & Chili

Servings: 2 Prep Time: 10 minutes

Cook Time: 15 minutes

1½ cups full-fat coconut milk

1½ cups filtered water or light veggie broth

1 stalk lemongrass, bruised & cut into 3–4 pieces

1 cup mushrooms (shiitake or oyster), sliced

1 cup chopped bok choy

1-inch piece fresh ginger, sliced thin

1 small red chili, sliced

1 tsp coconut aminos or tamari (optional, low-sodium)

Juice of ½ lime

Pinch sea salt

Optional: Thai basil or cilantro for garnish

1. Simmer the Aromatics

In a saucepan, combine coconut milk, water/broth, lemongrass, ginger, and chili.

Bring to a gentle simmer for 5–7 minutes, allowing flavors to infuse.

(Do not boil or the coconut milk may separate.)

2. Add mushrooms and bok choy. Simmer 5–6 more minutes, until mushrooms are tender and bok choy is just wilted.

3. Finish the Soup

Remove lemongrass pieces.

Stir in lime juice, coconut aminos (if using), and sea salt to taste.

Optional: add a splash of flax oil or a pinch of turmeric for extra anti-inflammatory depth.

To Serve

Ladle into bowls. Garnish with Thai basil, cilantro, or microgreens.

Optionally serve with a side of black rice or teff flatbread.

Za'atar-Crusted Trout with Roasted Carrots & Quinoa-Tahini Pilaf

Servings: 2 Prep Time: 15 minutes

Cook Time: 20 minutes

For the trout:

2 trout fillets (skin-on, \~4–5 oz each)

1½ tbsp za'atar (no added salt)

1 tsp olive oil

Pinch sea salt (optional)

For the roasted carrots:

3 medium carrots, sliced diagonally

1 tsp olive oil

¼ tsp ground cumin

Pinch sea salt

For the quinoa-tahini pilaf:

½ cup quinoa (rinsed)

1 cup water

1 tbsp tahini

Juice of ½ lemon

1 tbsp chopped parsley (optional)

Pinch sea salt

1. Roast the Carrots

Preheat oven to 400°F (200°C).

Toss carrots with olive oil, cumin, and sea salt.

Roast on a baking sheet for 20 minutes, flipping once halfway through.

2. Cook the Quinoa Pilaf

In a pot, combine quinoa, water, and salt. Bring to a boil.

Cover and simmer 15 minutes, or until water is absorbed.

Fluff and stir in tahini, lemon juice, and parsley.

3. Prepare the Trout

Pat trout fillets dry. Brush with olive oil and press za'atar onto flesh side.

Sear in a nonstick pan or grill skin-side down over medium heat for 3–4 minutes, then flip and cook **2–3 minutes** until cooked through.

Alternatively, bake at 375°F (190°C) for 10–12 minutes.

To Serve

Plate trout alongside roasted carrots and quinoa-tahini pilaf.

Optional garnish: lemon zest or sumac dusting for extra antioxidants.

Snacks and Treats

Golden Turmeric Tahini Bites with Black Pepper & Flaxseed

Servings: \10 small bites Prep Time: 10 minutes

¼ cup tahini (unsweetened, smooth)

2 tbsp ground flaxseed

1 tbsp date paste (or 1 soft Medjool date, mashed)

½ tsp ground turmeric

¼ tsp cinnamon

1 pinch freshly ground black pepper

Optional: 1 tsp shredded coconut or hemp seeds (for rolling)

1. Mix the Base

In a bowl, combine tahini, flaxseed, turmeric, cinnamon, and pepper.

Add date paste and stir until a thick dough forms. (Add a splash of warm water if too stiff.)

2. Form the Bites

Roll into \1-inch balls using your hands.

Optional: Roll in coconut or hemp seeds for texture.

3. Place in fridge for at least 15 minutes to firm up.

To Serve:

Enjoy as a functional snack or pre-meal blood sugar stabilizer.

Store in fridge (up to 5 days) or freezer (up to 2 weeks).

Frozen Wild Blueberry–Avocado Cups with Cacao Nibs

Servings: 6 small cups Prep Time: 10 minutes

Freeze Time: 2–3 hours

½ cup wild blueberries (frozen or fresh)

½ ripe avocado

¼ cup full-fat coconut cream (solid part only)

½ tsp vanilla extract (alcohol-free if possible)

1–2 tsp date paste or monk fruit

1 tbsp cacao nibs (for topping)

1. Blend the Base

In a small blender, combine blueberries, avocado, coconut cream, vanilla, and optional sweetener.

Blend until completely smooth.

2. Pour into Molds

Spoon mixture into silicone mini muffin molds or ice cube trays.

Tap lightly to remove air bubbles.

3. Sprinkle cacao nibs evenly over each cup.

4. Freeze

Freeze for 2–3 hours, or until solid.

Pop out and store in a freezer-safe container.

To Serve:

Let soften at room temperature for 2–3 minutes before eating.

Enjoy as an anti-inflammatory dessert or cooling afternoon snack.

Fermented Cashew Yogurt with Chia, Goji Berries & Cardamom

Servings: 2

Prep Time: 5 minutes (+ soaking time)

¾ cup unsweetened fermented cashew yogurt

2 tbsp chia seeds

2 tbsp dried goji berries (preferably soaked 10 mins)

¼ tsp ground cardamom

Optional: 1 tsp date paste or monk fruit (if more sweetness is desired)

1. Soak the Chia & Goji

In a small bowl, mix chia seeds with ¼ cup water.

Stir well and let sit for 10–15 minutes until gel-like.

Soak goji berries in warm water separately (optional for softness).

2. Assemble

In a bowl or jar, combine cashew yogurt, soaked chia, cardamom, and goji berries.

Mix gently until well combined.

3. Chill or Serve Immediately

Optional: Refrigerate for 30 minutes for flavors to meld.

Enjoy immediately or store refrigerated for up to 2 days.

To Serve:

Top with extra goji, hemp seeds, or crushed walnuts for texture & nutrient boost.

Perfect as an anti-inflammatory breakfast or gut-healing snack.

Roasted Spiced Pumpkin Seeds with Sumac & Nutritional Yeast

Servings: 4 snack portions Prep Time: 5 minutes

Cook Time: 12–15 minutes

1 cup raw pumpkin seeds (pepitas)

1½ tsp extra virgin olive oil

½ tsp sumac

1 tbsp nutritional yeast

¼ tsp smoked paprika

Small pinch sea salt (optional)

1. Preheat oven to 325°F (160°C). Line a baking sheet with parchment.

2. In a bowl, toss pumpkin seeds with olive oil, sumac, smoked paprika, and nutritional yeast until evenly coated.

3. Roast

Spread seeds in a single layer on baking sheet.

Roast for 12–15 minutes, stirring once halfway, until golden and crisp.

Let cool completely for max crunch.

To Serve:

Enjoy as a snack, salad topper, or sprinkle over roasted veggies or soups.

Store in an airtight jar for up to 1 week (or refrigerate for longer freshness).

Jicama Sticks with Avocado-Lime Dip & Microgreens

Servings: 2

Prep Time: 10 minutes

1 small jicama, peeled and cut into sticks

1 ripe avocado

Juice of 1 small lime

1 tsp extra virgin olive oil

Small pinch of sea salt (optional)

¼ cup fresh microgreens (broccoli, radish, or sunflower sprouts)

1. In a small bowl, mash avocado with lime juice, olive oil, and sea salt until smooth and creamy.

2. Peel and cut jicama into thin sticks or wedges for dipping.

3. Assemble & Serve

Spoon avocado dip into a serving bowl.

Top with fresh microgreens.

Serve with jicama sticks on the side.

To Serve:

Great as a fresh, cooling snack or appetizer.

Optional: add a pinch of ground cumin or chili flakes for a flavor boost.

Coconut-Collagen Matcha Bites with Spirulina & Macadamia

Servings: 10 small bites

Prep Time: 10 minutes

½ cup unsweetened shredded coconut

2 tbsp crushed raw macadamia nuts

1 tbsp hydrolyzed collagen powder (grass-fed)

1 tsp matcha powder

½ tsp spirulina powder

1 tsp raw honey (or ½ tsp if preferred less sweet)

1–2 tsp filtered water

1. In a bowl, combine coconut, macadamias, collagen, matcha, and spirulina.

2. Add Honey & Bind

Add honey and mix well.

Add 1–2 tsp of water slowly until mixture holds together when pressed.

3. Form Bites

Roll into small 1-inch balls or press into silicone molds.

Refrigerate for 15–20 minutes to firm.

To Serve:

Store in fridge (up to 5 days) or freezer (up to 2 weeks).

Ideal as an anti-inflammatory snack, workout fuel, or travel bite.

Baked Turmeric-Cauliflower Poppers with Smoky Paprika Dip

Servings: 2 Prep Time: 10 minutes

Cook Time: 25 minutes

For the cauliflower poppers:

2 cups cauliflower florets

1 tbsp extra virgin olive oil

½ tsp ground turmeric

½ tsp garlic powder

Pinch smoked paprika

Pinch sea salt

For the dip:

1 roasted red bell pepper (or use jarred, unsalted)

2 tbsp tahini

1 tsp lemon juice

¼ tsp smoked paprika

Pinch cumin (optional)

1. Bake the Cauliflower

Preheat oven to 400°F (200°C).

Toss cauliflower with olive oil, turmeric, garlic powder, paprika, and salt.

Spread on parchment-lined tray.

Roast for 20–25 minutes, flipping halfway, until golden and crisp at edges.

2. Blend the Dip

While cauliflower bakes, blend roasted pepper, tahini, lemon juice, paprika, and cumin until smooth.

Add a splash of warm water if needed for consistency.

To Serve

Serve warm cauliflower poppers with the smoky dip on the side or drizzled on top.

Optional: Garnish with parsley, crushed walnuts, or a sprinkle of hemp seeds.

Green Apple Nachos with Walnut-Cinnamon Spread

Servings: 2

Prep Time: 10 minutes (+ soaking time)

1 large green apple, thinly sliced

½ cup raw walnuts (soaked 4+ hours, drained)

½ tsp ground cinnamon

¼ tsp vanilla extract or powder

Small pinch sea salt

2 tsp hemp hearts (for topping)

1–2 tbsp filtered water (to blend)

1. Blend soaked walnuts with cinnamon, vanilla, salt, and 1–2 tbsp water until smooth and creamy (like a thick nut butter).

2. Slice apple thinly into rounds or wedges and lay them flat on a plate.

3. Assemble

Spoon or drizzle the walnut-cinnamon spread over the apple slices.

Sprinkle with hemp hearts.

To Serve

Serve immediately for best texture and flavor.

Optional: Add crushed freeze-dried raspberries or cacao nibs for extra antioxidant punch.

Raw Cacao–Lucuma Truffles with Brazil Nut Butter

Servings: \8 small truffles

Prep Time: 10 minutes

3 tbsp Brazil nut butter (or blend 4 Brazil nuts + 1 tbsp coconut oil)

1½ tbsp raw cacao powder

1 tbsp lucuma powder

¼ tsp Ceylon cinnamon

Small pinch sea salt

Optional: 1 tsp ground flaxseed or maca powder

1. Mix the Dough

In a bowl, combine Brazil nut butter, cacao, lucuma, cinnamon, and salt.

Mix until a thick, moldable dough forms.

If too dry, add a few drops of warm water or melted coconut oil.

2. Form Truffles

Roll into small 1-inch balls using your hands.

Optional: roll in extra lucuma, cacao powder, or shredded coconut.

3. Refrigerate for 15–20 minutes to firm up.

To Serve:

Store in fridge (up to 5 days) or freezer (2+ weeks).

Great as an anti-inflammatory dessert or selenium-boosting treat (1–2 max/day recommended due to selenium levels).

Seaweed Snack Rolls with Avocado, Kimchi & Toasted Sesame

Servings: 2 rolls (serves 1–2 as a snack)

Prep Time: 8–10 minutes

2 nori sheets

½ ripe avocado, mashed

¼ cup wild-fermented kimchi (drained slightly if very wet)

¼ cup cucumber, julienned or sliced thin

1 tsp toasted sesame seeds

Optional: dash of coconut aminos or a squeeze of lime

1. Lay & Layer

Place one nori sheet shiny side down on a clean surface.

Spread half the mashed avocado across the lower third.

Add a line of cucumber slices and a spoonful of kimchi.

Sprinkle with sesame seeds.

2. Roll It Up**

Gently roll up the nori sheet (like a sushi roll) from the bottom.

Seal the edge with a touch of water if needed.

Repeat for second roll.

3. Slice each roll in half or into bite-sized pieces using a sharp knife.

Soups and Stews

Miso–Seaweed Broth with Shiitake, Ginger & Bok Choy

Servings: 2 Prep Time: 10 minutes

Cook Time: 15 minutes

2 tbsp mellow white miso (unpasteurized)

3 cups filtered water or light vegetable broth

1 cup fresh shiitake mushrooms, sliced (or ½ cup dried, soaked)

1½ cups chopped bok choy

1-inch knob ginger, thinly sliced or grated

1 small sheet dried wakame or dulse (about 1 tbsp crumbled)

1 tsp toasted sesame oil or avocado oil (optional)

1 scallion, thinly sliced

1. Start the Broth

In a medium pot, heat water or broth over medium heat.

Add ginger and mushrooms. Simmer 10 minutes, until mushrooms are tender and broth is fragrant.

2. Add wakame and bok choy. Simmer 3–5 minutes, until greens are tender and seaweed rehydrated.

3. Turn off the heat. In a small bowl, mix miso with a bit of warm broth to thin it, then stir into the soup (do not boil miso to preserve probiotics).

4. Drizzle with sesame or avocado oil and top with sliced scallions.

To Serve:

Enjoy warm as a healing tonic or light meal.

Can be paired with a side of fermented vegetables or a spoon of hemp hearts for added omega-3s.

Sunchoke & Leek Soup with Fennel, Celery Root & Tarragon Oil

Servings: 3 Prep Time: 12 minutes

Cook Time: 20 minutes

For the Soup:

1 tbsp olive oil or avocado oil

1 medium leek (white/light green parts), sliced

1 cup fennel bulb, chopped

1½ cups sunchokes (Jerusalem artichokes), scrubbed and chopped

1 cup celery root (celeriac), peeled and diced

1 garlic clove, smashed (optional)

3 cups filtered water or vegetable broth

Pinch sea salt

For the Tarragon Oil:

1 tbsp chopped fresh tarragon

2 tbsp extra virgin olive oil

Pinch lemon zest (optional)

1. Sauté Aromatics

In a pot, heat oil over medium.

Add leeks, fennel, and garlic. Sauté 3–4 minutes, until softened but not browned.

2. Simmer the Veggies

Add sunchokes, celery root, water/broth, and salt.

Bring to a boil, reduce to low, and simmer 15–17 minutes, until all veggies are tender.

3. Blend the Soup

Let cool slightly, then blend until silky smooth (use immersion or upright blender).

Adjust thickness with more warm water if needed.

4. In a small bowl, stir tarragon into olive oil (with zest if using). Let infuse while soup blends.

To Serve:

Ladle soup into bowls. Drizzle with tarragon oil.

Optional: top with microgreens or crushed fennel seeds.

Golden Root Vegetable & Turmeric Coconut Stew

Servings: 3 Prep Time: 15 minutes

Cook Time: 25 minutes

For the Stew:

1 tbsp cold-pressed coconut oil

1 tsp grated fresh turmeric (or ½ tsp ground)

¼ tsp ground black pepper

1 clove garlic, minced

1 small red onion or shallot, finely chopped

1 cup sweet potato, peeled & cubed

1 cup carrot, sliced

1 cup parsnip, peeled & cubed

1 cup full-fat coconut milk

1½ cups filtered water or vegetable broth

Pinch sea salt

For the Cilantro Gremolata:

¼ cup chopped fresh cilantro

Zest of ½ lemon

1 tsp lemon juice

1 tsp cold-pressed olive oil

1. Sauté the Aromatics

In a pot, heat coconut oil over medium.

Add onion, garlic, turmeric, and black pepper. Sauté 2–3 minutes, until fragrant.

2. Stir in sweet potato, carrot, and parsnip. Toss for a minute to coat in spices.

3. Simmer the Stew

Pour in coconut milk and water/broth.

Bring to a boil, then reduce to low and simmer 20–25 minutes, until veggies are soft.

4. In a small bowl, combine cilantro, lemon zest, juice, and olive oil. Stir well.

To Serve:

Ladle stew into bowls and top with a spoonful of cilantro gremolata.

Optional: Add a few crushed toasted pumpkin seeds for crunch and zinc.

Smoky Tomato–Red Lentil Soup with Cumin

Servings: 3 Prep Time: 10 minutes

Cook Time: 20 minutes

1 tbsp extra virgin olive oil (plus more for drizzling)

1 small red onion, chopped

1 garlic clove, minced

1 tsp ground cumin

½ tsp smoked paprika

⅔ cup red lentils, rinsed

1½ cups chopped tomatoes (fresh or no-salt added canned)

2½ cups filtered water or vegetable broth

½ tsp sumac (plus more for topping)

Pinch sea salt

Optional: lemon zest or chopped parsley for garnish

1. Sauté Base Aromatics

Heat olive oil in a pot over medium.

Add onion and garlic, sauté 3–4 minutes, until softened.

Stir in cumin and paprika, cook 30 seconds more.

2. Simmer the Soup

Add red lentils, chopped tomatoes, and water/broth.

Bring to a boil, reduce to low heat.

Simmer uncovered for 15–18 minutes, until lentils are soft.

3. Blend (Optional)

Use an immersion blender for a creamy texture, or leave chunky.

Stir in sumac and salt to taste.

To Serve:

Ladle into bowls, drizzle with olive oil, sprinkle extra sumac.

Optional: top with lemon zest or parsley for brightness.

Broccoli & Cauliflower Bisque

Servings: 3 Prep Time: 10 minutes (+ optional soaking)

Cook Time: 15 minutes

For the Bisque:

1 tbsp olive oil or avocado oil

1 small leek or onion, chopped

2 cups broccoli florets

2 cups cauliflower florets

2½ cups water or light vegetable broth

1 garlic clove (optional)

Pinch sea salt

Squeeze of lemon juice (for brightness)

For the Lemon-Zest Cashew Cream:

⅓ cup raw cashews (soaked 2 hrs or boiled 5 min)

¼ cup filtered water

Zest of ½ lemon

1 tsp lemon juice

Pinch sea salt

1. Sauté the Base

Heat oil in a pot over medium.

Add leeks/onions and garlic (if using), cook 3–4 minutes until translucent.

2. Cook the Veggies

Add broccoli, cauliflower, and water/broth.

Simmer 10–12 minutes, until vegetables are tender but not overcooked.

3. Blend the Bisque

Let cool slightly, then blend until silky smooth (immersion or upright blender).

Stir in a squeeze of lemon juice and pinch of salt.

4. Blend soaked cashews with water, lemon zest, lemon juice, and salt until smooth.

To Serve:

Ladle bisque into bowls. Swirl in lemon-zest cashew cream.

Optional: top with microgreens, hemp seeds, or steamed broccoli florets.

Spiced Okra & Black-Eyed Pea Stew with Fenugreek

Servings: 3 Prep Time: 12 minutes

Cook Time: 25 minutes

1 tbsp cold-pressed avocado or olive oil

1 tsp fenugreek seeds

1 small red onion, chopped

1 clove garlic, minced

1 cup fresh or frozen okra, sliced

1 cup cooked black-eyed peas (or canned, rinsed)

1 tsp ground coriander

½ tsp turmeric

1½ cups water or light vegetable broth

1 tbsp tamarind paste (unsweetened)

Pinch sea salt

1. Bloom the Spices

Heat oil in a pot over medium.

Add fenugreek seeds and let them sizzle for 30–45 seconds.

Stir in onion and garlic, sauté 3–4 minutes until softened.

2. Add Vegetables & Simmer

Add okra, black-eyed peas, coriander, turmeric, and salt.

Stir for a minute to coat, then pour in water/broth.

Simmer 15–18 minutes, until okra is tender and stew slightly thickened.

3. Finish with Tamarind

Stir in tamarind paste and simmer for 2–3 minutes more.

Adjust salt and thickness as needed.

To Serve:

Serve warm in a bowl, optionally topped with chopped fresh parsley or cilantro.

Pairs beautifully with a spoon of fermented millet or warm sautéed amaranth greens.

Wild Mushroom & Root Vegetable Stew with Thyme

Servings: 3 Prep Time: 15 minutes

Cook Time: 30 minutes

1 tbsp olive or avocado oil

1 small leek or shallot, chopped

2–3 cloves black garlic, mashed

1½ cups wild mushrooms (shiitake, maitake, oyster), sliced

1 cup carrot, diced

1 cup rutabaga or turnip, peeled and cubed

1 cup parsnip or sweet potato, peeled and cubed

3 cups vegetable broth or filtered water

1 tsp dried thyme (or 1 tbsp fresh)

Pinch sea salt

Optional: 1 tsp grated fresh ginger

1. Sauté Aromatics & Mushrooms

Heat oil in a soup pot over medium.

Add leek and sauté 2–3 minutes.

Stir in black garlic, mushrooms, and thyme. Cook 5–6 minutes, until mushrooms soften and begin to brown.

2. Add Root Veggies & Simmer

Add carrots, rutabaga, and parsnip (or sweet potato). Stir well.

Pour in broth, bring to a boil, then reduce heat.

Simmer 20–25 minutes, until all vegetables are tender and stew thickens naturally.

3. Finish & Adjust

Add salt to taste. Stir in optional ginger if using.

Let rest covered for 5 minutes off heat to allow flavors to deepen.

To Serve:

Serve in bowls, optionally garnished with a drizzle of olive oil and fresh thyme leaves.

Pairs well with a spoon of fermented root kraut or hemp seed crumble on top.

Nettle–Green Pea Soup with Mint

Servings: 2–3 Prep Time: 10 minutes

Cook Time: 10 minutes

1 tbsp olive oil or avocado oil

1 small shallot or leek, chopped

1 cup fresh or frozen green peas

1–1½ cups fresh nettle leaves (rinsed, tough stems removed)

1 tbsp fresh mint leaves (or ½ tsp dried)

Juice of ½ lemon + zest (optional)

2½ cups filtered water or light vegetable broth

2 tbsp hemp seeds (for garnish)

Pinch sea salt

1. Sauté Aromatics

In a pot, heat oil over medium.

Add shallot/leek and sauté 2–3 minutes until translucent.

2. Simmer Veggies

Add green peas, nettles, and mint.

Pour in water or broth, bring to a simmer.

Cook 5–7 minutes, just until peas and nettles are tender.

3. Blend the Soup

Let cool slightly, then blend until smooth (immersion or upright blender).

Stir in lemon juice, zest (if using), and salt to taste.

To Serve:

Ladle into bowls. Sprinkle each serving with 1 tbsp hemp seeds.

Optional: drizzle with extra virgin olive oil or swirl in unsweetened coconut yogurt for extra creaminess.

Chickpea & Carrot Tagine with Cinnamon

Servings: 3 Prep Time: 10 minutes

Cook Time: 25 minutes

- 1 tbsp olive oil or avocado oil
- 1 small red onion, finely chopped
- 1 garlic clove, minced
- 1 tsp ground turmeric
- ½ tsp ground cinnamon
- 1 cup carrots, sliced into coins
- 1½ cups cooked chickpeas (or 1 can, rinsed)
- ¼ cup dried apricots, chopped
- 1½ cups filtered water or low-sodium vegetable broth
- Pinch sea salt
- Optional: 1 tsp fresh lemon juice (to finish)
- Optional garnish: fresh parsley or slivered almonds

1. Sauté Aromatics

In a medium pot or tagine base, heat oil over medium.

Add onion and garlic, cook 3–4 minutes, until soft.

Stir in turmeric and cinnamon, toast spices for 30 seconds.

2. Add Veggies & Simmer

Add carrots, chickpeas, and chopped apricots.

Pour in broth/water and bring to a gentle boil.

Reduce heat and simmer uncovered 15–20 minutes, until carrots are soft and sauce has slightly thickened.

3. Add salt to taste and a splash of lemon juice if desired.

To Serve:

Serve warm over quinoa, millet, or cauliflower mash.

Top with parsley or toasted slivered almonds for added minerals.

Thai Lemongrass & Coconut Soup with Mushrooms

Servings: 2–3 Prep Time: 10 minutes

Cook Time: 15 minutes

1½ cups full-fat coconut milk

1 cup filtered water or light veggie broth

2 stalks lemongrass, smashed and chopped into large pieces

3 lime leaves (fresh or dried)

1 cup mushrooms (shiitake, oyster, or button), sliced

1–2 small red chilies, sliced (adjust to heat tolerance)

1-inch fresh ginger or galangal, sliced thin

Juice of 1 lime

½ tsp sea salt or to taste

Optional garnish: chopped fresh cilantro or Thai basil

1. Simmer the Aromatics

In a pot, combine coconut milk, water/broth, lemongrass, lime leaves, ginger, and chili.

Bring to a gentle simmer (not a full boil) for 5–7 minutes to infuse flavors.

2. Add sliced mushrooms and cook another 5–7 minutes, until mushrooms are soft but not overcooked.

3. Finish & Strain (Optional)

Remove lemongrass and lime leaves if desired.

Stir in lime juice and salt to taste.

To Serve:

Ladle into bowls, garnish with cilantro or Thai basil.

Optional: add a swirl of chili oil or top with a few hemp seeds for omega-3s.

Low FODMAP Options

Zucchini Noodles with Gingered Carrot Sauce

Servings: 2 Prep Time: 10 minutes

Cook Time: 10 minutes

Base:

2 medium zucchinis (spiralized)

2 tbsp pine nuts (toasted in dry pan)

Carrot-Ginger Sauce:

1 cup chopped carrots

1-inch knob fresh ginger (grated)

1 tbsp cold-pressed olive oil or avocado oil

¼ cup water (or as needed)

Pinch of sea salt

Optional Enhancements:

½ tsp lemon zest

1 tsp basil oil (or finely chopped fresh basil + olive oil)

1. Make the Sauce

Steam or boil carrots until soft (8–10 minutes).

Blend with ginger, oil, and water until smooth. Add salt to taste. Thin as needed for pourable consistency.

2. Spiralize zucchini. If desired, lightly sauté for 1–2 minutes in a dry or lightly oiled pan to soften — or leave raw for more crunch.

3. Assemble

Toss zucchini noodles with warm carrot-ginger sauce.

Top with toasted pine nuts.

Finish with lemon zest and a drizzle of basil oil (optional but powerful).

To Serve:

Serve immediately as a light lunch or pair with grilled anti-inflammatory protein (sardines, tofu, or hempseed patty).

Grilled Salmon with Lemon-Herb Ghee

Servings: 2 Prep Time: 10 minutes

Cook Time: 10 minutes

For the salmon:

2 wild salmon fillets (\5 oz each)

1 tsp olive oil (for grill or pan)

Pinch sea salt

Lemon-Herb Ghee:

1½ tbsp grass-fed ghee

1 tsp lemon zest

1 tsp finely chopped parsley or dill

Optional: pinch of turmeric or black pepper

Salad:

1 cup arugula

1 cup watercress

1 tbsp pumpkin seeds (lightly toasted)

¼ cup microgreens (any type)

1 tsp olive oil

1 tsp lemon juice

1. Make Lemon-Herb Ghee

In a small pan, gently warm ghee until melted (do not brown).

Stir in lemon zest, herbs, and optional turmeric. Set aside.

2. Grill the Salmon

Preheat grill or skillet to medium-high.

Lightly oil and season salmon with sea salt.

Grill skin-side down for 4–5 minutes, flip and cook another 3–4 minutes or until flaky.

3. Toss the Salad

Combine arugula, watercress, pumpkin seeds, and microgreens in a bowl.

Drizzle with olive oil and lemon juice just before serving.

To Serve:

Plate grilled salmon and spoon lemon-herb ghee over top.

Serve salad alongside or underneath salmon for a nutrient-packed one-plate meal.

Steamed Japanese Pumpkin (Kabocha)

Servings: 2 Prep Time: 10 minutes

Cook Time: 15–18 minutes

2 cups kabocha squash (peeled & cubed, \1-inch pieces)

For the sauce:

½ cup full-fat coconut milk

¾ tsp ground turmeric (or 1½ tsp fresh, grated)

½ tsp grated fresh ginger

1 tsp cold-pressed coconut oil

Pinch sea salt

Optional: pinch of black pepper

Garnish (optional but powerful):

1 tsp toasted coconut flakes

½ tsp lime zest

1. Steam the Kabocha

Place squash cubes in a steamer basket over boiling water.

Cover and steam for 12–15 minutes, or until fork-tender.

2. Make the Coconut-Turmeric Sauce

In a small saucepan, combine coconut milk, turmeric, ginger, coconut oil, and sea salt.

Warm gently over low heat for 2–3 minutes, stirring occasionally. Don't boil.

3. Assemble

Plate steamed kabocha and drizzle with warm coconut-turmeric sauce.

Finish with lime zest and/or toasted coconut flakes if using.

To Serve:

Serve as a side dish or anti-inflammatory plant-based light meal.

Pairs well with a spoon of fermented daikon or a warm quinoa bowl.

Fennel & Cucumber Salad with Dill Oil

Servings: 2 Prep Time: 10 minutes

For the Salad:

1 medium fennel bulb, thinly sliced

1 small cucumber, thinly sliced (peeled if desired)

Pinch sea salt

Dill-Lemon Oil Dressing:

2 tbsp extra virgin olive oil

1 tsp finely chopped fresh dill (or ½ tsp dried)

½ tsp lemon zest

1 tsp lemon juice

Optional Protein Add-On:

½ cup firm tofu or tempeh, sliced

1 tsp olive or avocado oil (for searing)

Pinch sea salt + turmeric (optional)

1. In a small bowl, whisk olive oil, dill, lemon zest, and lemon juice. Set aside.

2. Assemble the Salad

Toss fennel and cucumber with a pinch of sea salt.

Drizzle with dill-lemon oil and let sit for 5 minutes to soften slightly.

3. Optional Protein (if using)

Heat oil in a non-stick pan over medium.

Lightly sear tofu or tempeh slices for 2–3 minutes per side.

Optional: Dust with turmeric while searing for an extra anti-inflammatory boost.

To Serve

Plate salad and top with warm tofu or tempeh (if using).

Garnish with fennel fronds or extra dill.

Crispy Baked Eggplant Slices with Miso-Free Romesco

Servings: 2 Prep Time: 15 minutes

Cook Time: 25 minutes

For the Eggplant:

1 medium eggplant, sliced into ¼-inch rounds

1 tbsp garlic-infused olive oil

1 tbsp ground flaxseed (optional, helps crisp)

Pinch sea salt

Optional: 1 tsp smoked paprika or dried thyme

For the Romesco Sauce:

1 medium roasted red bell pepper (peeled)

2 tbsp blanched almonds (lightly toasted)

1 tbsp garlic-infused olive oil

½ tsp smoked paprika

1 tsp lemon juice

Pinch sea salt

Optional: 1 tbsp water (to thin, if needed)

1. Prepare & Bake Eggplant

Preheat oven to 400°F (200°C).

Brush both sides of eggplant slices with garlic-infused oil.

Sprinkle with sea salt, optional flaxseed, and paprika or thyme.

Arrange on parchment-lined tray.

Bake 12–15 minutes, flip, then another 8–10 minutes until golden and crisping.

2. Make Miso-Free Romesco

In a blender or food processor, combine red pepper, almonds, garlic-infused oil, lemon juice, paprika, and salt.

Blend until smooth; thin with a bit of water if needed for a spoonable sauce.

To Serve

Plate eggplant slices and drizzle or dip with romesco sauce.

Garnish with chopped parsley or crushed pumpkin seeds for crunch.

Bok Choy & Ginger Soup with Carrots

Servings: 2 Prep Time: 10 minutes

Cook Time: 15 minutes

4 cups filtered water or low-FODMAP vegetable broth

2 baby bok choy (sliced lengthwise or chopped)

1 medium carrot, julienned or thinly sliced

1½ tsp grated fresh ginger

¾ cup cooked rice noodles (or \70g dry, pre-soaked)

½ cup oyster mushrooms, sliced (optional)

1 tbsp coconut aminos or tamari (gluten-free)

1 tsp cold-pressed sesame or avocado oil

Juice of ½ lime

Optional garnish: lime zest, cilantro, or sliced scallion greens

1. Simmer the Base

In a pot, bring water or broth to a light boil.

Add grated ginger, carrots, and mushrooms (if using). Simmer 5 minutes.

2. Add Bok Choy & Noodles

Add bok choy and pre-soaked or par-cooked rice noodles.

Simmer another 4–5 minutes, just until greens are tender and noodles are soft.

3. Finish with Flavor

Stir in coconut aminos/tamari and sesame oil.

Remove from heat, add fresh lime juice just before serving.

To Serve

Ladle into bowls.

Top with lime zest, cilantro, or scallion greens if desired.

Serve warm and enjoy gut-soothing comfort in every spoonful.

Crispy Skin Chicken Thighs with Roasted Japanese Eggplant

Servings: 2 Prep Time: 15 minutes

Cook Time: 30–35 minutes

For the chicken:

2 skin-on, bone-in pastured chicken thighs

1 tsp garlic-infused olive oil

Pinch sea salt + black pepper (optional)

½ tsp turmeric or smoked paprika (optional)

For the vegetables:

1 Japanese eggplant, halved lengthwise

2 large carrots, peeled and chopped

1 tbsp garlic-infused olive oil

Sea salt to taste

Optional: splash of lemon juice or apple cider vinegar

1. Prep the Chicken

Preheat oven to 400°F (200°C).

Pat chicken skin dry. Rub with garlic-infused oil, salt, and optional turmeric or paprika.

Place skin-side down in a cold oven-safe skillet. Turn heat to medium-high and sear for **5–6 minutes** until skin crisps.

Flip and transfer skillet to oven. Roast for 18–20 minutes, until fully cooked (165°F/74°C internal).

2. Roast the Eggplant & Carrots

On a separate baking sheet, toss eggplant and chopped carrots in garlic-infused oil and a pinch of sea salt.

Roast alongside chicken for 20–25 minutes, flipping halfway.

Remove eggplant when golden and soft; continue roasting carrots if needed for purée.

3. Blend roasted carrots with a splash of warm water, optional lemon juice, and a pinch of salt. Blend until smooth.

To Serve

Spoon carrot purée onto plate.

Place crispy chicken thigh on top.

Add roasted eggplant on the side.

Optional: garnish with fresh thyme or parsley.

Grilled Zucchini & Parsnip Skewers

Servings: 2 Prep Time: 15 minutes

Cook Time: 12–15 minutes

1 medium zucchini, sliced into thick half-moons

1 medium parsnip, peeled & sliced into thin rounds or batons

1 tbsp garlic- or chive-infused olive oil

1 tbsp finely chopped fresh chives

Pinch sea salt

Optional: splash of lemon juice or lemon zest

1. Steam or boil parsnips for 4–5 minutes until slightly tender. Drain and cool.

2. Assemble the Skewers

Alternate zucchini and parsnip slices on soaked wooden or metal skewers.

Brush lightly with infused olive oil and sprinkle with sea salt.

3. Grill the Skewers

Preheat grill or grill pan to medium-high.

Grill skewers for 10–12 minutes, turning occasionally, until veggies are golden and tender.

4. Finish with Chives

Drizzle with a little more infused olive oil and sprinkle fresh chives over the top.

Optional: add lemon zest or juice just before serving.

To Serve

Serve hot as a main veggie feature or side.

Pairs beautifully with grilled wild fish, seared firm tofu, or a lentil-based dip.

Low-FODMAP Couscous with Riced Celeriac

Servings: 2 Prep Time: 10 minutes

Cook Time: 5–6 minutes

1 cup peeled celeriac, riced or finely grated

½ cup carrot, riced or grated

2 tbsp finely chopped flat-leaf parsley

1 tsp ground sumac

1 tsp garlic-infused olive oil

Pinch sea salt

Optional: squeeze of lemon juice

1. Grate or food-process the celeriac and carrot into fine, couscous-like texture.

2. Sauté Briefly

In a non-stick or ceramic skillet, heat garlic-infused olive oil over medium.

Add riced celeriac and carrot with a pinch of salt.

Sauté for 4–5 minutes, just until slightly softened but not mushy.

3. Finish & Season

Remove from heat. Stir in parsley, sumac, and optional lemon juice.

Let cool slightly to let the flavors meld.

To Serve:

Serve warm or at room temp as a base or side.

Protein Add-ons:

4–6 grilled shrimp per serving, or

1 soft- or hard-boiled egg per person

Chia & Pumpkin Seed Crackers with Coconut Yogurt Dip

Servings: \30 crackers + dip for 2 Prep Time: 10 minutes

Cook Time: 35–40 minutes (crackers)

For the Chia–Pumpkin Seed Crackers:

½ cup ground pumpkin seeds (or pumpkin seed meal)

¼ cup whole chia seeds

¼ cup ground flaxseed

¼ tsp sea salt

½ cup water

Optional: 1 tsp rosemary or thyme (dried)

For the Coconut Yogurt Dip:

½ cup plain unsweetened coconut yogurt

1 tbsp garlic- or chive-infused olive oil

1 tbsp chopped fresh parsley or dill

½ tsp lemon zest

Pinch of sea salt

1. Make the Cracker Dough

In a bowl, mix pumpkin seed meal, chia, flaxseed, salt, and herbs (if using).

Add water and stir to form a gel-like dough. Let sit for 10 minutes to thicken.

2. Bake the Crackers

Preheat oven to 325°F (160°C).

Spread dough thinly (⅛ inch) on a parchment-lined tray.

Score into squares with a knife or pizza cutter.

Bake for 35–40 minutes, flipping once if needed, until crisp and golden.

3. In a small bowl, stir yogurt with infused oil, herbs, lemon zest, and sea salt. Chill until ready to serve.

To Serve:

Break crackers apart and serve with herbed yogurt dip.

Optional: add microgreens or a few thin slices of radish for texture.

Beverages and Liquid Diet Options

Ginger-Turmeric Bone Broth Elixir

Servings: 1 Prep Time: 3 minutes

Heat Time: 5 minutes

1½ cups high-quality bone broth (preferably grass-fed or pastured)

1 tsp freshly grated turmeric (or ½ tsp ground)

1 tsp freshly grated ginger (or ½ tsp ground)

1 tsp MCT oil (start with ½ tsp if new to it)

Juice of ½ lemon (about 1 tbsp)

Pinch of sea salt or mineral salt

Optional: black pepper

1. In a small saucepan, gently heat bone broth over medium-low — avoid boiling to preserve amino acids.

2. Whisk in turmeric, ginger, and sea salt. Simmer gently for 2–3 minutes.

3. Remove from heat. Stir in lemon juice and MCT oil. Add black pepper if using.

4. For a frothy, emulsified drink, blend for 10 seconds on low speed.

To Serve:

Sip warm, ideally on an empty stomach in the morning, or during a gut rest window.

Cucumber–Celery Juice with Parsley & Aloe Vera

Servings: 1

Prep Time: 5 minutes

- 1 large cucumber (peeled if waxed)
- 2 celery stalks (organic preferred)
- ¼ cup flat-leaf parsley (lightly packed)
- 2 tbsp aloe vera gel (from inner leaf only, no latex)
- ¼ cup cold filtered water (to thin, optional)
- Optional: a squeeze of lime or pinch of mineral salt

1. Prepare Ingredients

Wash all produce thoroughly.

Roughly chop cucumber and celery for blending or juicing.

Use inner gel only from aloe leaf (or pure bottled inner leaf gel).

2. Juice or Blend

Juicer method: Run cucumber, celery, and parsley through juicer. Stir in aloe gel afterward.

Blender method: Blend all ingredients + water until smooth. Strain through a fine mesh sieve or nut milk bag.

3. Serve immediately for maximum enzyme activity. Can be chilled for up to 12 hours.

To Use:

Ideal first thing in the morning or between meals for gut reset.

Gentle enough for IBS, gastritis, or leaky gut support.

Blueberry–Camu Camu Smoothie with Hemp Milk & Chia Gel

Servings: 1

Prep Time: 5 minutes

(Chia gel can be made in advance)

Ingredients:

¾ cup unsweetened hemp milk

1 tbsp chia seeds (pre-soaked in 3 tbsp water for 10–15 min to make gel)

1 cup frozen wild blueberries (or fresh if available)

½ tsp camu camu powder (start with ¼ tsp if new to it)

½ small frozen banana (optional – adds texture, low histamine)

1 tsp flaxseed oil or 1 tbsp hemp seeds

1. Combine 1 tbsp chia seeds with 3 tbsp water. Let sit 10–15 min until gelled.

2. Blend

Add all ingredients to blender: hemp milk, chia gel, blueberries, camu camu, and banana (if using).

Blend until smooth and creamy.

3. Taste & Adjust

Add more hemp milk if thinner texture is preferred.

Sweeten lightly (optional) with ½ medjool date or monk fruit if needed.

To Serve:

Drink immediately for maximum antioxidant activity.

Can be chilled or frozen into smoothie pops for skin flare-up days.

Warm Dandelion Root Latte with Ceylon Cinnamon

Servings: 1 Prep Time**: 3 minutes

Cook Time: 5 minutes

1 cup filtered water

1 tbsp roasted dandelion root (loose or 1 tea bag)

¼ tsp Ceylon cinnamon (not cassia)

2 tbsp full-fat coconut cream (no additives)

Optional: ½ tsp raw monk fruit, date syrup, or vanilla powder

1. Brew the Dandelion Root

Bring water to a light simmer.

Add dandelion root. Simmer for 3–4 minutes (or steep 5–7 min if using tea bag).

2. Strain & Blend

Strain tea into a heat-proof blender.

Add cinnamon, coconut cream, and optional sweetener. Blend for 15–20 seconds until frothy.

(Or whisk vigorously in a saucepan to emulsify.)

3. Reheat gently to desired temperature without boiling.

To Serve:

Sip slowly, ideally morning or evening on an empty or light stomach.

Especially useful during fasting windows, PCOS flares, or after heavy meals.

Spiced Golden Milk with Black Pepper, Cardamom

Servings: 1 Prep Time: 2 minutes

Cook Time: 5 minutes

1 cup unsweetened almond, coconut, or hemp milk

½ tsp ground turmeric (or 1 tsp fresh grated)

⅛ tsp ground cardamom (or 2 crushed pods)

⅛ tsp ground cinnamon (optional)

Pinch of black pepper

½ tsp ashwagandha powder (root extract)

1 tsp coconut oil or MCT oil

Optional: monk fruit, date syrup, or a slice of fresh ginger

1. Warm the Milk

In a small saucepan, heat milk over low-medium heat.

Add turmeric, cardamom, cinnamon (if using), and black pepper.

2. Simmer & Stir

Whisk gently while warming for 3–5 minutes, ensuring spices dissolve.

Turn off heat and stir in ashwagandha powder and coconut oil (if using).

3. Blend for 10 seconds for a smooth, creamy consistency, or use a frother.

To Serve:

Sip slowly in the evening or during stress recovery, PMS, or chronic fatigue episodes.

Best taken 30–60 minutes before bed for adaptogenic effect.

Green Mineral Broth with Kelp, Nettles & Ginger

Servings: \4 cups Prep Time: 10 minutes

Cook Time: 45 minutes (simmer)

1 cup loosely packed fresh nettle leaves (or 1 tbsp dried)

1 strip dried kombu or 1 tsp powdered kelp

1-inch piece of fresh ginger, sliced

1 stalk celery, chopped

1 small zucchini, chopped

1 handful spinach or parsley

4 cups filtered water

Pinch of mineral salt (or leave unsalted for fasting use)

1. Combine & Simmer

Add all ingredients to a medium pot with water.

Bring to a light boil, then reduce to low heat.

Simmer gently for 40–45 minutes uncovered.

2. Strain or Blend

Strain to use as a clear sipping broth.

OR blend (with added hemp or avocado) into a green soup.

3. Optional Add-Ins (post-cook)

1 tsp lemon juice or ACV

1 tbsp hemp oil or flaxseed oil

Dash cayenne or turmeric for added inflammation modulation

To Use:

Drink warm in the morning, between meals, or during detox/fasting phases.

Acts as a nourishing base for soups or medicinal smoothies.

Coconut Water with Lime Juice, Mint & Chia Seeds

Servings: 1 Prep Time: 2 minutes

Soaking Time: 10 minutes (for chia)

1 cup pure coconut water (unsweetened)

Juice of ½ fresh lime

1 tbsp chia seeds

4–5 mint leaves (lightly bruised)

Optional: pinch of mineral salt or crushed ice

1. Soak Chia

In a glass, stir chia seeds into coconut water.

Let sit for 10–15 minutes, stirring once midway, until gel forms.

2. Add Flavor

Stir in lime juice and mint leaves (bruise lightly to release oils).

Add salt if desired for extra electrolytes.

3. Enjoy immediately, or refrigerate for up to 8 hours. Stir well before sipping.

To Use:

Ideal post-workout, on flights, during illness, or after gut flares.

Can be sipped between meals or alongside light anti-inflammatory meals.

Raw Cacao & Reishi Mushroom Smoothie

Servings: 1

Prep Time: 5 minutes

¾ cup unsweetened almond or hemp milk

½ small ripe avocado

1 tbsp raw cacao powder

½ tsp Ceylon cinnamon

½ tsp reishi mushroom powder (dual-extract preferred)

1 tsp hemp seeds or flax oil (for omega-3s)

Optional: ½ frozen banana (gentle sweetness), monk fruit, or ½ date

Optional: pinch of sea salt or vanilla powder

1. Blend

Add all ingredients to a high-speed blender.

Blend for 30–45 seconds, until creamy and smooth.

Adjust liquid for thinner consistency if needed.

2. Add more cacao for bitterness, cinnamon for spice, or sweetener if needed.

To Use:

Perfect as a nutrient-dense breakfast, post-fast liquid meal, or evening adrenal support tonic**.

Can be served chilled or gently warmed (without boiling) for a latte-like feel.

30-DAY ANTI-INFLAMMATORY MEAL PLAN

Day 1

- Morning: Ginger-Turmeric Bone Broth Elixir — p.158
- Breakfast: Buckwheat-Kale Pancakes — p.105
- Lunch: Black Garlic & Wild Salmon over Teff Polenta — p.94
- Snack: Golden Turmeric Tahini Bites — p.125
- Dinner: Sunchoke & Leek Soup with Parsley Oil — p.98

Day 2

- Morning: Cucumber–Celery Juice with Parsley & Aloe — p.159
- Breakfast: Fermented Cashew Yogurt with Chia, Goji & Cardamom — p.127
- Lunch: Charred Eggplant, Lentil & Za'atar-Stuffed Collard Wraps — p.106
- Snack: Roasted Spiced Pumpkin Seeds with Sumac — p.128
- Dinner: Lotus Root & Adzuki Bean Stir-Fry — p.108

Day 3

- Morning: Warm Dandelion Root Latte with Cinnamon & Coconut Cream — p.161
- Breakfast: Blueberry–Camu Camu Smoothie with Hemp Milk & Chia Gel — p.160
- Lunch: Golden Beet, Arugula & Hemp Heart Salad — p.107
- Snack: Jicama Sticks with Avocado-Lime Dip — p.129
- Dinner: Shiitake Mushroom & Bok Choy Hotpot — p.101

Day 4

- Morning: Green Mineral Broth with Kelp, Nettles & Ginger — p.163
- Breakfast: Amaranth-Crusted Tempeh with Braised Cabbage — p.120
- Lunch: Green Papaya & Avocado Salad — p.102
- Snack: Coconut-Collagen Matcha Bites with Spirulina — p.130
- Dinner: Okra, Quinoa & Fermented Lemon Stew — p.99

Day 5

- Morning: Spiced Golden Milk with Black Pepper, Cardamom — p.162
- Breakfast: Buckwheat Noodles with Charred Broccoli — p.116
- Lunch: Sardine-Nori Lettuce Wraps with Avocado — p.96
- Snack: Raw Cacao–Lucuma Truffles with Brazil Nut Butter — p.133
- Dinner: Broccoli & Cauliflower Bisque — p.140

Day 6**

- Morning: Raw Cacao & Reishi Mushroom Smoothie — p.165
- Breakfast: Miso-Braised Turnips & Shiitake Mushrooms — p.112
- Lunch: Golden Beet & Arugula Salad with Hemp Seeds — p.119
- Snack: Chia & Pumpkin Seed Crackers with Coconut Yogurt Dip — p.156
- Dinner: Wild Mushroom & Root Vegetable Stew with Thyme — p.142

Day 7

- Morning: Coconut Water with Lime Juice, Mint & Chia Seeds — p.164
- Breakfast: Bok Choy & Ginger Soup with Carrots — p.152
- Lunch: Artichoke & Turmeric-Fennel Chickpea Cakes — p.95
- Snack: Baked Turmeric-Cauliflower Poppers — p.131
- Dinner: Grilled Sardines w/ Stewed Tomatoes & Millet — p.111

Day 8

- Morning: Ginger–Turmeric Bone Broth Elixir — p.158
- Breakfast: Sunchoke & Asparagus Stir-Fry with Cumin — p.121
- Lunch: Chaga-Infused Wild Rice Pilaf — p.103
- Snack: Golden Turmeric Tahini Bites — p.125
- Dinner: Chickpea & Carrot Tagine with Cinnamon — p.144

Day 9

- Morning: Cucumber–Celery Juice with Parsley & Aloe Vera — p.159
- Breakfast: Fermented Cashew Yogurt with Chia, Goji & Cardamom — p.127
- Lunch: Fennel & Cucumber Salad with Dill Oil — p.150
- Snack: Jicama Sticks with Avocado-Lime Dip — p.129
- Dinner: Thai Coconut Soup w/ Lemongrass, Bok Choy & Chili — p.122

Day 10

- Morning: Spiced Golden Milk with Cardamom & Black Pepper — p.162
- Breakfast: Carrot-Ginger Soup with Coconut & Red Lentils — p.115
- Lunch: Stuffed Collard Wraps with Quinoa — p.114
- Snack: Raw Cacao–Lucuma Truffles — p.133
- Dinner: Smoky Tomato–Red Lentil Soup with Cumin — p.139

Day 11

- Morning: Coconut Water w/ Lime Juice, Mint & Chia Seeds — p.164
- Breakfast: Buckwheat-Kale Pancakes — p.105
- Lunch: Sunchoke & Leek Soup with Fennel, Celery Root & Tarragon Oil — p.137
- Snack: Roasted Spiced Pumpkin Seeds with Sumac — p.128
- Dinner: Grilled Salmon with Lemon-Herb Ghee — p.148

Day 12

- Morning: Raw Cacao & Reishi Mushroom Smoothie — p.165
- Breakfast: Miso–Seaweed Broth with Shiitake, Ginger & Bok Choy — p.136
- Lunch: Eggplant & Tomato Tagine with Chickpeas — p.118
- Snack: Coconut-Collagen Matcha Bites — p.130
- Dinner: Thai Lemongrass & Coconut Soup with Mushrooms — p.145

Day 13

- Morning: Cucumber–Celery Juice with Aloe & Parsley — p.159
- Breakfast: Amaranth-Crusted Tempeh with Braised Cabbage — p.120
- Lunch: Green Papaya & Avocado Salad — p.102
- Snack: Seaweed Snack Rolls with Avocado, Kimchi & Toasted Sesame — p.134
- Dinner: Spiced Okra & Black-Eyed Pea Stew w/ Fenugreek — p.141

Day 14

- Morning: Warm Dandelion Root Latte — p.161
- Breakfast: Bok Choy & Ginger Soup with Carrots — p.152
- Lunch: Shiitake Mushroom & Bok Choy Hotpot — p.101
- Snack: Chia & Pumpkin Seed Crackers + Coconut Yogurt — p.156
- Dinner: Wild-Caught Salmon with Roasted Purple Cauliflower — p.113

Day 15**

- Morning: Green Mineral Broth with Nettles, Kelp & Ginger — p.163
- Breakfast: Golden Root Vegetable & Turmeric Coconut Stew — p.138
- Lunch: Golden Beet, Arugula & Hemp Heart Salad — p.107
- Snack: Baked Turmeric-Cauliflower Poppers — p.131
- Dinner: Wild Mushroom & Root Vegetable Stew — p.142

Day 16

- Morning: Ginger–Turmeric Bone Broth Elixir — p.158
- Breakfast: Turmeric-Infused Lentil Soup — p.110
- Lunch: Smoked Mackerel, Kohlrabi & Beet Slaw — p.100
- Snack: Golden Turmeric Tahini Bites — p.125
- Dinner: Sunchoke & Leek Soup with Parsley Oil — p.98

Day 17

- Morning: Blueberry–Camu Camu Smoothie — p.160
- Breakfast: Buckwheat Noodles with Charred Broccoli — p.116
- Lunch: Artichoke & Turmeric-Fennel Chickpea Cakes — p.95
- Snack: Raw Cacao–Lucuma Truffles — p.133
- Dinner: Broccoli & Cauliflower Bisque — p.140

Day 18

- Morning: Spiced Golden Milk — p.162

- Breakfast: Carrot-Ginger Soup w/ Coconut & Red Lentils — p.115
- Lunch: Lotus Root & Adzuki Bean Stir-Fry — p.108
- Snack: Jicama Sticks with Avocado-Lime Dip — p.129
- Dinner: Grilled Sardines w/ Stewed Tomatoes & Millet — p.111

Day 19

- Morning: Coconut Water with Lime & Mint — p.164
- Breakfast: Thai Lemongrass & Coconut Soup — p.145
- Lunch: Chaga-Infused Wild Rice Pilaf — p.103
- Snack: Coconut-Collagen Matcha Bites — p.130
- Dinner: Charred Eggplant, Lentil & Za'atar-Stuffed Collards — p.106

Day 20

- Morning: Raw Cacao & Reishi Smoothie — p.165
- Breakfast: Miso-Braised Turnips & Shiitake Mushrooms — p.112
- Lunch: Fennel & Cucumber Salad with Dill Oil — p.150
- Snack: Golden Turmeric Tahini Bites — p.125
- Dinner: Thai Coconut Soup w/ Lemongrass & Chili — p.122

Day 21

- Morning: Dandelion Root Latte — p.161
- Breakfast: Buckwheat-Kale Pancakes — p.105
- Lunch: Golden Beet, Arugula Salad with Hemp — p.119
- Snack: Roasted Spiced Pumpkin Seeds — p.128
- Dinner: Eggplant & Tomato Tagine w/ Chickpeas — p.118

Day 22

- Morning: Cucumber–Celery Juice — p.159
- Breakfast: Sunchoke & Asparagus Stir-Fry — p.121
- Lunch: Green Papaya & Avocado Salad — p.102
- Snack: Seaweed Snack Rolls w/ Kimchi — p.134
- Dinner: Nettle–Green Pea Soup with Mint — p.143

Day 23

- Morning: Spiced Golden Milk — p.162
- Breakfast: Golden Root Vegetable & Coconut Stew — p.138
- Lunch: Black Lentil & Pomegranate Molasses Bowl — p.97
- Snack: Raw Cacao–Lucuma Truffles — p.133
- Dinner: Crispy Skin Chicken Thighs with Roasted Eggplant — p.153

Day 24

- Morning: Green Mineral Broth — p.163
- Breakfast: Bok Choy & Ginger Soup — p.152

- Lunch: Stuffed Collard Wraps with Quinoa — p.114
- Snack: Baked Turmeric-Cauliflower Poppers — p.131
- Dinner: Miso–Seaweed Broth with Bok Choy — p.136

Day 25

- Morning: Coconut Water with Chia & Lime — p.164
- Breakfast: Okra, Quinoa & Fermented Lemon Stew — p.99
- Lunch: Smoked Mackerel, Kohlrabi & Beet Slaw — p.100
- Snack: Chia & Pumpkin Seed Crackers — p.156
- Dinner: Golden Cauliflower & Broccoli Stir-Fry — p.104

Day 26

- Morning: Cucumber–Celery Juice — p.159
- Breakfast: Thai Lemongrass Soup — p.145
- Lunch: Charred Eggplant Collard Wraps — p.106
- Snack: Coconut-Collagen Matcha Bites — p.130
- Dinner: Za'atar-Crusted Trout with Carrots & Quinoa Pilaf — p.123

Day 27

- Morning: Dandelion Latte — p.161
- Breakfast: Amaranth-Crusted Tempeh — p.120
- Lunch: Golden Beet & Arugula Salad — p.119
- Snack: Roasted Pumpkin Seeds — p.128
- Dinner: Sunchoke & Leek Soup with Parsley Oil — p.98

Day 28

- Morning: Coconut Water with Lime & Mint — p.164
- Breakfast: Buckwheat Noodles w/ Charred Broccoli — p.116
- Lunch: Chaga-Infused Wild Rice Pilaf — p.103
- Snack: Golden Turmeric Tahini Bites — p.125
- Dinner: Spiced Okra & Black-Eyed Pea Stew — p.141

Day 29

- Morning: Raw Cacao & Reishi Smoothie — p.165
- Breakfast: Broccoli & Cauliflower Bisque — p.140
- Lunch: Sardine-Nori Lettuce Wraps — p.96
- Snack: Jicama Sticks with Avocado-Lime Dip — p.129
- Dinner: Wild-Caught Salmon with Purple Cauliflower — p.113

Day 30

- Morning: Spiced Golden Milk — p.162
- Breakfast: Zucchini Noodles with Gingered Carrot Sauce — p.147
- Lunch: Fennel & Cucumber Salad with Dill Oil — p.150

- Snack: Raw Cacao–Lucuma Truffles — p.133
- Dinner: Wild Mushroom & Root Vegetable Stew — p.142

RECIPE INDEX

Recipe Title	Page
Amaranth-Crusted Tempeh with Braised Cabbage	120
Artichoke & Turmeric-Fennel Chickpea Cakes	95
Baked Turmeric-Cauliflower Poppers with Smoky Paprika Dip	131
Black Garlic & Wild Salmon over Teff Polenta with Dandelion Greens	94
Black Lentil & Pomegranate Molasses Bowl	97
Blueberry-Camu Camu Smoothie with Hemp Milk & Chia Gel	160
Bok Choy & Ginger Soup with Carrots	152
Broccoli & Cauliflower Bisque	140
Buckwheat Noodles with Charred Broccoli	116
Buckwheat-Kale Pancakes	105
Carrot-Ginger Soup with Coconut & Red Lentils	115
Charred Eggplant, Lentil & Za'atar-Stuffed Collard Wraps	106
Chaga-Infused Wild Rice Pilaf	103
Chia & Pumpkin Seed Crackers with Coconut Yogurt Dip	156
Chickpea & Carrot Tagine with Cinnamon	144
Coconut Water with Lime Juice, Mint & Chia Seeds	164
Coconut-Collagen Matcha Bites with Spirulina & Macadamia	130
Crispy Baked Eggplant Slices with Miso-Free Romesco	151
Crispy Skin Chicken Thighs with Roasted Japanese Eggplant	153
Cucumber-Celery Juice with Parsley & Aloe Vera	159
Dandelion Root Latte with Ceylon Cinnamon & Coconut Cream (Warm)	161
Eggplant & Tomato Tagine with Chickpeas	118
Fermented Cashew Yogurt with Chia, Goji Berries & Cardamom	127
Fennel & Cucumber Salad with Dill Oil	150
Frozen Wild Blueberry-Avocado Cups with Cacao Nibs	126

Ginger-Turmeric Bone Broth Elixir with MCT & Lemon	158
Golden Beet & Arugula Salad with Hemp Seeds	119
Golden Beet, Arugula & Hemp Heart Salad	107
Golden Cauliflower & Broccoli Stir-Fry	104
Golden Root Vegetable & Turmeric Coconut Stew	138
Golden Turmeric Tahini Bites with Black Pepper & Flaxseed	125
Grilled Salmon with Lemon-Herb Ghee	148
Grilled Sardines with Stewed Tomatoes, Olives & Fennel over Millet	111
Grilled Zucchini & Parsnip Skewers	154
Green Apple Nachos with Walnut-Cinnamon Spread	132
Green Mineral Broth with Kelp, Nettles & Ginger	163
Green Papaya & Avocado Salad	102
Jicama Sticks with Avocado-Lime Dip & Microgreens	129
Lotus Root & Adzuki Bean Stir-Fry	108
Miso-Seaweed Broth with Shiitake, Ginger & Bok Choy	136
Miso-Braised Turnips & Shiitake Mushrooms	112
Nettle-Green Pea Soup with Mint	143
Okra, Quinoa & Fermented Lemon Stew	99
Raw Cacao & Reishi Mushroom Smoothie with Avocado & Cinnamon	165
Raw Cacao-Lucuma Truffles with Brazil Nut Butter	133
Roasted Brussels Sprouts & Grapes	117
Roasted Spiced Pumpkin Seeds with Sumac & Nutritional Yeast	128
Sardine-Nori Lettuce Wraps with Avocado	96
Seaweed Snack Rolls with Avocado, Kimchi & Toasted Sesame	134
Shiitake Mushroom & Bok Choy Hotpot	101
Smoky Tomato-Red Lentil Soup with Cumin	139
Smoked Mackerel, Kohlrabi & Beet Slaw	100
Spiced Golden Milk with Black Pepper, Cardamom & Ashwagandha	162
Spiced Okra & Black-Eyed Pea Stew with Fenugreek	141
Steamed Japanese Pumpkin (Kabocha)	149
Stuffed Collard Wraps with Quinoa	114
Sunchoke & Asparagus Stir-Fry with Cumin	121

Sunchoke & Leek Soup with Fennel, Celery Root & Tarragon Oil	137
Sunchoke & Leek Soup with Parsley Oil	98
Thai Coconut Soup with Lemongrass, Mushrooms, Bok Choy & Chili	122
Thai Lemongrass & Coconut Soup with Mushrooms	145
Turmeric-Infused Lentil Soup with Mustard Seeds & Coconut Milk	110
Wild Mushroom & Root Vegetable Stew with Thyme	142
Wild-Caught Salmon with Roasted Purple Cauliflower	113
Za'atar-Crusted Trout with Roasted Carrots & Quinoa-Tahini Pilaf	123
Zucchini Noodles with Gingered Carrot Sauce	147

Made in United States
Cleveland, OH
11 July 2025